Right Use of Power: The Heart of Ethics

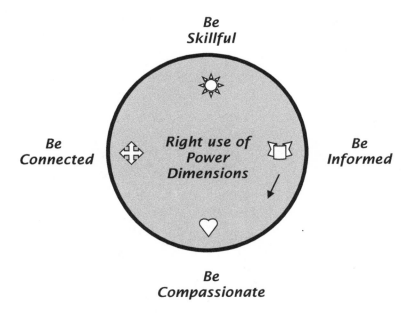

Be
Skillful

Be
Connected

Right use of
Power
Dimensions

Be
Informed

Be
Compassionate

Dr. Cedar Barstow,
M.Ed., C.H.T., D.P.I.

A Guide and Resource for Professional Relationships

Right Use of Power: The Heart of Ethics

A guide and resource
for those in professional positions
of service and trust, e.g.:

Psychotherapists
Massage Therapists
Social Workers
Bodyworkers
Physicians
Teachers
Leaders
Clergy
Nurses
Coaches
Counselors
Consultants

For information about
resources and books, free newsletter
Workshops, CE courses, and Teacher's Training go to:
www.rightuseofpower.org

Copyright ©2005 by Cedar Barstow
10th Anniversary Edition, 2015
Many Realms Publishing
Boulder, Colorado

ISBN#: 978-0-9743746-8-0

Cover by Richard Barrett
Photo by Dr. Reynold Feldman

Endorsements

"I know of nothing quite like this book. It offers a wealth of useful, exquisitely organized information. A valuable resource; it is a book which both informs and delights. On the subject of ethics, it can't be topped."
Ron Kurtz,
Author of "Body-Centered Psychotherapy: The Hakomi Therapy"

"Cedar Barstow has written the best book I've seen on the ethics, dangers, and potentials inherent within helping relationships. This is the book I wish I had read when I was first training as a psychotherapist.
Bill Plotkin,Ph.D.
Author of "Soulcraft: Crossing into the Mysteries of Nature and Psyche"

"This is an outstanding resource guide. It is comprehensive, clear, inspirational, and practical. A great contribution to a shift in ethics education."
Angeles Arrien, Ph.D.
Author of "The Four-Fold Way" and "Signs of Life"

The Right Use of Power by Cedar Barstow teaches ethics from the inside out. Most ethics courses for psychotherapists teach us the laws and scare us into using them. The approach of this book and the trainings based on it help people graduate to a deeper connection to their own ethical natures, an internal sense of their own integrity, and a personal view of what is right in their relations with clients. This is much more interesting and helpful than memorizing legal statutes. Wonderfully experiential and deeply didactic, I consider it my favorite book for teaching ethics in the field of psychotherapy.
Rob Fisher, MFT,
Author of "Experiential Psychotherapy with Couples:
A Guide for the Creative Pragmatist"

Cedar has culminated in her book years of her work in teaching ethics to professionals and in living these ethics on personal, community and professional and political levels. She is precise, descriptive, and graphic in her charts, her examples, and applications of ethical issues. She elevates the entire discussion of ethical issues far above a philosophy of "avoiding legal issues," to a philosophy of service with highest of regard for humanity and the processes that facilitate a higher moral ground.
Laura S. Dodson, M.S.W., Ph.D., Jungian Analyst,
Author of "Virginia Satir: Her Life and Circle of Influence"

Cedar's work is so 'right' for our times. She embodies the principles she teaches in her work and empowers others to do the same. Dedicated to the growth of the human spirit in relationship, she has produced both a book and home study course that will help individuals, groups and organizations make quantum leaps in their capacity to live the potential of love and trust in our human associations. I recommend her approach with heartfelt warmth and deep appreciation.

Mukara Meredith, MSW,
President, Matrix Leadership Consultants

Right Relations is a concept that ought to be foundational for living the interdependent web of world community. Wise and accountable use of power is central to Right Relations. Cedar beautifully invites and instructs us in this journey that is both personal and internal as well as communal.

Rev. Dr. Marni Harmony
Unitarian Universalist Minister

The ethical conduct of professional relationships is a complicated and delicate subject. This book tackles it in as clear and sensitive a way as I've seen. I highly recommend it.

Richard C. Schwartz, Ph.D.
Author of "Internal Family Systems"

Responses from Readers:

"I am having fun. I wish I had nothing else to do but the course. A remarkable job has been done collecting all this information, establishing it within a spiritual and healing orientation, and then making it so easily accessible and experiential."

"My whole idea of professional ethics was broadened and deepened through seeing ethics in the larger context of right use of power. Personally, I studied my relationship with power, my wounds around power, and how I use power. This was engaging, surprising, and helpful. I now have an increased awareness of the more subtle ways in which power and influence are exercised."

"I see that ethics is pro-active, not just about knowing what not to do. I see that it's never too late to repair and get re-connected after a conflict or misunderstanding."

Camille Leaver, psychotherapist

"I found the book to be extremely invigorating. In studying other texts, I could actually feel my body tense up and become anxious due to the 'constrictions' being focused on. With a relationship-prudent view, I can now focus my helping attention more effectively."

Bob Graham, outdoor leadership guide

"Even though the program is for helping professionals, I find that in my everyday life, I experience both power and influence, from all directions, and sometimes, even with the best of intentions, I misuse both. Becoming aware of the ethics behind power and influence is so helpful in being more aware of my interactions."

Chia-Tzn

"In pastoral training we talk about something we call the ministry of presence. The presence you teach is akin to this. It is the attentive heart staying present to a situation regardless of the efficacy of words or actions. Your work gives me a felt sense of the healing environment that is created through a heart-centered understanding of power."

Sue Cummings
Manager of Pastoral Care, Waterford Hospital

"You speak eloquently about how clients just want to know that you can be trusted—no sleight of hand, no deception, no grandiose technique is needed."

Mary Seamster, Watsu practitioner

Who this book is for:

The theory and ideas put forth here are intended to be of inspiration and practical guidance and support for caregivers in all helping professions. Because the author is a body psychotherapist and thus most familiar with this modality, the wording often refers to therapists. Other professional descriptors include: practitioners, caregivers, healers, body workers, counselors, teachers, physicians, nurses, clergy, coaches, and consultants. The information for psychotherapists and social workers is valuable and readily translatable to other care-giving relationships. Understanding the values, responsibilities and dynamics of role power differences is essential. Reframing ethics as power with heart is a significant shift. It brings compassion to power and power to compassion.

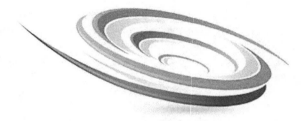

RIGHT USE OF POWER
INSTITUTE

Right Use of Power Workshops

For current information on national and international workshops
Go to: www.RightUseofPower.org
- o   taught by Dr. Cedar Barstow
- o   taught by trained Right Use of Power teachers

Workshops provide a personally engaging and insightful format for increasing ethical awareness and wisdom in the use of power with heart. Augment and increase your understanding and integration of the material in this book by attending a workshop. Find out more about the curriculum and workshop opportunities by clicking on Workshops at the website.

Right Use of Power Teacher Trainings

For current information on national and international trainings
Go to: www.rightuseofpower.org

The Teacher's Training is an additional 2-4 day training with follow-up activities to prepare you to present the Right Use of Power approach in your own programs, be listed as a teacher on the website, and join the Right Use of Power Teacher's Guild. All Teacher Trainings are taught by Cedar Barstow or Senior Trainers. Find out more about the curriculum, resources and opportunities available to teachers by clicking on Workshops at the website.

Right Use of Power E-Courses

This book can be used for Continuing Education Credit (CE Hours) for many professions. Find all the details at our website.

Go to: www.rightuseofpower.org

Resources

Our website has many resources: free monthly newsletter, free materials, other books, articles, and international RUP teacher listing. Use the search tool to access articles and blogposts that update or expand on the topics in this book.

Go to: www.rightuseofpower.org

Ethics with Wisdom and Power with Heart

Introduction to this 10th Anniversary Edition

What an honor to find that the material in this book has withstood the test of time! So, I don't need to write a new book, just add some pieces to the book I wrote in 2005.

Over the last 10 years hundreds of people have read the book, taken related workshops, consulted with me, completed e-courses, subscribed to my newsletter, and/or trained to be Right Use of Power teachers. To all these people I offer my gratitude for their insightful ideas and refining feedback. Sections that have been added or expanded include those on power differential, ethics and technology, status power, relationship between hierarchy and equality, saying yes to and owning up- and down-power roles, using down-power influence, leadership styles, the shadow side of power, power parameters, forgiveness, making an effective apology, risk management, and grievance processes. In the added 100 pages, you will find additional depth and complexity.

Internet technology provides some immeasurable gifts. Through the Right Use of Power Institute website (**www.rightuseofpower.org**) you will be able to find out more about topics in the book and also keep up with new ideas and developments. Just go to the website and click on the search tool. Entering any topic will take you to related articles and blog posts. Given its universal nature, Right Use of Power material should not become dated. At our website you can also sign up for our newsletter and look for workshops, teachers, and ways to get involved.

The Right Use of Power ethics approach has grown over the past 20 years from an idea to a book to a series of books and now to an Institute with teachers, resources, multiple programs, a website, continuing-education offerings, an office, and an Administrative Director. This development has been a richly rewarding collaborative effort. I want to appreciate and acknowledge Amanda Mahan, the Institute's current Administrative Director and the creative, wise, devoted technological wizard who has built an artistic website and infrastructure for the Right Use of Power Institute (RUPI). She is also talented teacher as well as a mentor to new Right Use of Power teachers. She blesses me with her strong, compassionate ability to work things out. What joy, moreover, to have the constant love and support of my extraordinary husband, Reynold Ruslan "Ren" Feldman. He stretches my vision with big, expansive ideas and stays around with his feet on the ground as a business consultant, fundraiser, writer, editor, and kind, loving soul and companion. He co-authored the Right Use of Power book for lay people: *Living in the Power Zone: How Right Use of Power Can Transform Your Relationships* (2014). My Hakomi colleague Magi Cooper has contributed significant ideas and processes; she is now also teaching Right Use of Power teacher trainings. Warm, funny, wise, skillful and full of integrity, Magi buoys me up. Magi and Peg Syverson now join me as co-trainers in RUP.

I wish to recognize and thank members of the RUPI Board of Directors, particularly Marni Harmony, Chair, Cliff Penwell, and Richard Ireland for their insightful and generous advice; Doug McLean for editing the new sections; Judith Blackburn, Amina Knowlan, Shelley Tanenbaum, and Mukara Meredith for good, challenging conversations and input. Gratitude and appreciation go to all the Right Use of Power Guild Members, especially those who have been actively teaching Right Use of Power programs and integrating its ideas and processes into their work with groups such as psychotherapists, bodyworkers, students, massage therapists, youth, small-business leaders, and coaches. They have been forging new paths and helping ever larger groups of people understand and reframe their beliefs about ethics, power, conflict, shame and feedback. These individuals include Kathy Ginn, Vinay Gunther, Michael Moore, Sabrina Kindell, Rebecca Lincoln, Peg Syverson, Kathleen O'Rourke, Fenna Diephuis, Carrie Thomas Scott, Richard Ireland, Susan Buckles, Deena Martin, Ellen Palme, David Medema, Amanda Mahan, Magi Cooper, Louise Broomberg, Sallie Ingle, Julia Corley, Charna Rosenholtz, Natalie Collins, Jenny Morawska, Margaret Bassal, Conway Weary, Jonathan Macintyre, Joyce Ellenbecker, Kate Burns, Connie Burns, Wendy Crosman, Laurie Adato, Kippi Klausen, Eva Fajardo, and Athina Davies, Regina Smith, Jeff Coulliard, and all the other Advanced Teachers.

Welcome to this enhanced, highly revised and enriched 10th-anniversary edition of *Right Use of Power—The Heart of Ethics*. I hope you will find ideas and techniques here that will be useful in both your personal and your professional lives.

Cedar Barstow, M.Ed., CHT
Boulder, Colorado
July 2015
(minor edit and update) May 2018

I often ask people to express how they are different or work differently as a result of what they have learned through Right Use of Power training. Here are some representative responses:

- I will take better care of myself.
- I will practice engaging my curiosity in difficult situations.
- I will actively notice my impact.
- I will lean in to conflict with more skill.

- I will remember the image of the scarf for putting on and taking off the power that goes with my up- power roles.
- I will be more ethically pro-active.
- I will ask and not assume.
- I will see the positive potential in down-power roles.

- I will be more aware of the shadow aspects of power.
- I will campaign for the idea that power is not awful and that the power differential serves a valuable purpose.
- I will make sure to stay in the feedback loop.
- I will be more transparent in my thinking and decision-making.

- I will acknowledge and use my moral compass.
- I feel clearer about my power shadow and how to mediate it.
- I will bring in more balance between strength and compassion.
- I will be bold when I feel it is needed.

- I will own my power, both personal and role, and say a full "yes."
- I will use the four dimensions of power in so many situations.
- I will track for relationship disconnects instead of avoiding them.
- I will continue to engage myself with the theme of power.

RIGHT USE OF POWER PLEDGE

I pledge to use my personal and professional power with strength and heart. I will endeavor to stay connected, accountable, sensitive and skillful. I know that my right uses of power will help prevent and repair harm, resolve conflict and promote well being.

SIGNATURE

RIGHT USE OF POWER INSTITUTE
WWW.RIGHTUSEOFPOWER.ORG

Table of Contents

Dimension Three: Be Connected

Dimension Four: Be Skillful

Foreword

I have known Cedar Barstow since 1985 as a teacher, friend and colleague. It has been a privilege to write The Foreword for this outstanding book on the "Right Use of Power," as it is written by a woman about whom I can say for certain, "Cedar walks her talk."

It is more than timely that a book such as this becomes available to caregivers and students who are hungry for a new perspective on how to prevent and deal with the misuse of power. Her experiential approach invites our higher conscience to punch in and get to work, as Cedar begins to wake up readers to their inner ethical master. She calls us to be cognizant of all the ways we have consciously or unconsciously misused our power, or have had power misused against us. However, this book does not just leave us wounded and bleeding over these unfortunate events. For, Cedar offers methods that go deep enough to heal the festering wounds that have resulted when power has been misused, or when power has not been embraced; when it could have helped.

Power is a subject that conjures up images of dictators, regulatory agencies, malpractice suits, corporate misconduct, terrorist acts and ethics judgments. No wonder we have an automatic reflex to play Ostrich when the signs of moral discontent are coming our way! The cultural scenario of power as "rules and abuse" is neutralized when Cedar lays out her definition of power: "Power is the capacity or potential to bring change." Hearing this description reveals a relieving and shining paradigm: Ethics can be reparative instead of punitive.

After this refreshing shift, Cedar proceeds to pick the dusty locks on the doors of our inner storage bins, where we encounter our own wrathful deities who tell us in a loud voice, "Don't go there!!" Then, in a soothing, gentle tone, she invites these sentinels to step back. Surprisingly they do, and there in the cob-webbed corners of memory banks, the former abuses of power that we have been ashamed to tell anyone, (even our supervisors) begin to emerge. With these exiles unburdened and brought to the light; Cedar offers partner exercises that provide ways to heal from the feelings stuffed in the "shame-event dungeon," and be welcomed back by our compassionate colleagues, and our own forgiving Self. This transformational chapter concludes with a list of self-initiated stages that can help us with owning, letting go, learning and healing from shame-driven events.

Cedar invites us to embrace our natural compassionate awareness and become truthful with ourselves and with others. For as we cruise down the highway of good intentions, there are detours, and we may take a wrong turn. We all get lost from time to time. She believes that many grievances have their roots in the following postulate: "Our impact may be different than our intention." When you think deeply about this simple statement, it begins to illuminate some uncomfortable truths. Cedar has that way of guiding your light.

One of the many kaleidoscopes that shift one's consciousness in this book are the stories. This is an interactive book with stories that evoke recognitions that make us realize that we have all been there, ready to admit it or not. And been there in a similar way to those who offered their amazing tales. The stories themselves, in their candidness, inspire a sweet compassion for all who have suffered from abuses of power.

In one chapter, Cedar gives you the full monty about what actually happens when a complaint is filed to a licensure board against a therapist. This is like encountering Excalibur in your living room! The reader can't believe this woman is so fearlessly ranting about a subject that is rarely approached without judgment, force and fear (which usually makes you only skim or skip the reading). She has you so conditioned to not react by this point in the book, that you actually read this! And, you are riveted.

After the "what really happens in a complaint," she outlines statistics gathered from one state in the USA—Colorado. These fascinating statistics reveal the judgments that the Colorado Grievance Board made on all the complaints in one given year. It is relieving, revealing, sometimes surprising; and not as big a deal as our fears made them out to be. This unfolds against a backdrop of material that instructs the reader on how to track and contact the subtle relationship shifts in your clients long before they escalate. She discusses practical ways to repair rifts before they turn into grievances. She patiently explains that because of the power differential, it is the therapist's job to reconnect with the client or to suggest mediation. As you paddle the murky waters of transference and counter-transference, this book can be a guiding light.

Cedar recommends ways to mediate conflicts and to take responsibility for your 150% of the power differential. Though there are some instances when it is clear that a license should be revoked; (e.g., sexual contact between therapist and client); many lesser complaints should never have had to be heard in a grievance process. They could have been mediated long before the hurt and anger took them to the never-never land of ethics boards. This book gives you the tools to avoid that unthinkable event.

Cedar puts a calming hand on the finger that is ready to press the automatic button that connects to your attorney, and lets you know that there is another path. She encourages you to calm your ego and enter into the heart of darkness, in order to find your true heart again. For relationship is what we really want, and when it is fractured, in Cedar's mind, we can do a lot to begin to connect again. This book restores to the student some important long lost qualities of true Self: courage, compassion, connection and conscience. It points the way to climb another rung of the ladder of moral development. You cannot read "Right Use of Power" and not be changed.

Barbara Cargill M.A., A.D.T.R., C.H.T
Boulder, Colorado

The most common way people give up their power is by thinking they don't have any.
Alice Walker

There is guidance for each of us, and by lowly listening we shall hear the right word. . . .Place yourself in the middle of the stream of power and wisdom that flows into your life.
Ralph Waldo Emerson

My life belongs to the whole community, as long as I live it is my privilege to do for it whatever I can. I want to be thoroughly used up when I die...When you make somebody else do something against their will, that, to me, is not power. That is force. To me, force is a negation of power...By power I mean—almost exclusively—the ability to empower.
George Bernard Shaw[i]

When the generativity and responsiveness of our power is guided by loving concern for the well-being of all, we will have an ethical and sustainable world. Power directed by heart. Heart infused with power. This is the key to right use of power.   *CB*

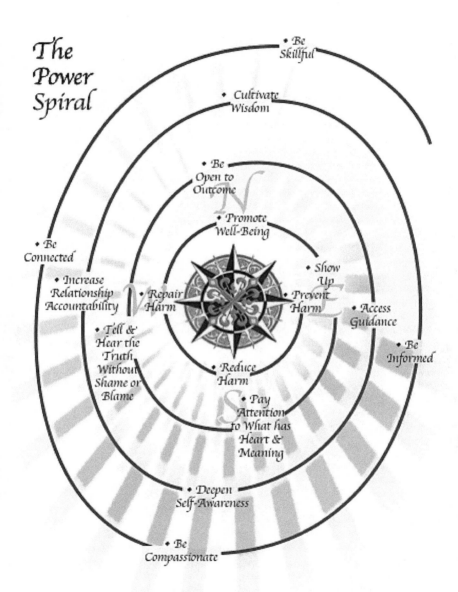

The
Power
Spiral

• Be
Skillful

• Cultivate
Wisdom

• Be
Open to
Outcome

• Promote
Well-Being

• Be
Connected

• Increase
Relationship
Accountability

• Repair
Harm

• Show
Up

• Prevent
Harm

• Access
Guidance

• Be
Informed

• Tell &
Hear the
Truth
Without
Shame or
Blame

• Reduce
Harm

• Pay
Attention
to What has
Heart &
Meaning

• Deepen
Self-Awareness

• Be
Compassionate

Power and Heart

The "Right Use of Power and Influence" is one of the most crucial needs of our time and one of the greatest challenges we face in leadership arenas as well as in personal development. Using power in an ethical way is learning to use power wisely. The ability to sustain relationship with skill and wisdom in the face of challenging ethical issues is power with heart. We have the capacity for wisdom in our use of power, yet we have been wounded by misuses and abuses of power by those in positions of trust. We have also inevitably misused or under-used our power in professional and personal situations.

Power is simply the ability to have an effect, or to have influence. However, the right use of this influence is complex. The right use of power in positions of trust is not simply the result of good intentions. It is also the ability to act sensitively, creatively, and effectively in the service of others and yourself. This requires engaging attention, relationship mastery, and a lifetime involvement in increasing sensitivity to the impact of our use of power.

The greatest revolutions science has presented to us across history point to a fundamental revolution of spirit and ethic equally profound, waiting in the wings.
Joseph P. Firmage[ii]

We need an ethic of compassion more desperately than ever before.
Karen Armstrong[iii]

The fundamental shift in ethics that is advocated here brings together power and heart. We have been conditioned to think that we need to choose between heart and power. Of ultimate importance in ensuring mutual well-being and resolving conflict, this shift is hinged on ownership and full use of our personal and professional power. The Right Use of Power method engages compassion and teaches us to stay related through conflict and to repair relationships. By revising our ideas about power, we begin to embody an ethic that includes both power and heart. This heartful ethic builds peace with dignity, and truth with compassion, and strength with vulnerability.

Be Skillful

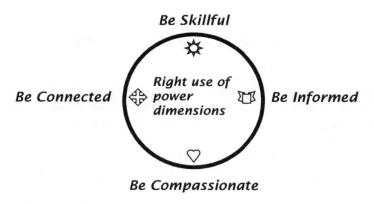

Be Connected   **Be Informed**

Be Compassionate

Human beings are capable of magnificent acts of wisdom, compassion, self-correction, and courage. We are capable of using power for healing, for connecting, and for peacemaking. Helping professionals often speak of their yearning for the satisfaction of finding a heartful power and using it to make real their altruistic intentions. Right Use of Power supports and builds on this desire. The Right Use of Power approach is a curriculum for the deepening of compassion, sensitivity, and the ability to resolve problems. This is ethics and power understood from a deep inner place that knows the value of staying connected.

Excess baggage

It seems that most of us carry "extra baggage" in our associations with both "ethics" and "power." Ethics, sadly, is often associated with such things as imposed rules, shame and blame, litigation, and self-righteousness. Power has been primarily associated with force, domination, abuse, and humiliation. To reframe power and ethics in ways that can be effective we need to discover, name, and release conditioned beliefs. Ethics in the context of the right use of power and its influence engages and heightens our awareness of the many impacts of the professional power differential and allows us to have time to feel nourished by our own integrity and desire to be in right relationship.

A young woman was constantly "on her own case." In her perception, nothing she did was ever good enough. When she finished one thing, she started right in on the next thing on her list with no pause for satisfaction or for recognizing her accomplishments and the goodness of her intentions. *She described succeeding in working out a significant issue with her roommate, and without taking a breath, began talking about something else that wasn't working. The leader asked her to stop for a moment. "Wait, you did something effective and courageous. Let's take a little time to acknowledge this and let yourself feel nourished by your success." She replied, "But I really want to work on that stuff about my body image." The leader said, "There'll be time for that, but good things need attention too. Let's do something to mark this moment. Let's light this little candle while we take a pause. You can take the candle with you and light it to recognize other moments of feeling good about yourself." There were tears flowing down her cheeks. "No one has ever acknowledged me for anything but good grades. This is so important and good."* In the Right Use of Power approach, we honor and acknowledge our innate goodness and desire to serve. We move from power-blindness to power intelligence.

Definitions

Here are a few working definitions

Ethics— a dictionary definition says that ethics is the study of what is right and wrong and of duty and moral obligation. For our purpose, ethics is a set of values, attitudes, and skills intended to have benevolent effects when applied through professional behavioral guidelines, decision-making processes, and the practice of compassion.

Power—most simply, is the ability to act or to have an effect. It is what enables us to do things. ***Influence*** is how we interact with others to make changes and have an effect. ***Role Power*** is the increased power that accompanies a professional role. This is called the ***power differential***. ***Personal power*** is the generative capacity to use our gifts and make real our intentions.

Compassion—resonating concern, an ability to see and respond to the connection between everyone and everything[iv].

Power Spiral—visual model for practicing right use of power in a multi-layered continuum.

Right Use of Power—the use of personal and role power and influence to prevent, reduce, resolve, and repair harm, and in addition, to balance and integrate strength with heart, improve relationships and situations, and promote well-being and the common good. *(In this context it is understood that power itself is neutral meaning that it can be used to bring harm or well-being depending on consciousness, skill, and intention. The use of the word 'right" is not meant to imply a black and white concept of right vs. wrong or good vs. evil.)*

Foundational Values

In affirming Right Use of Power as the heart of ethics, we are framing ethics and power in a very comprehensive way. These values form the foundation for the Right Use of Power approach.

Aspirational

We begin by acknowledging our desire and capacity for magnificence in the use of our personal and professional power. Supporting and engaging this desire accesses the "social engagement system." According to the work of Stephen Porges,[v] this third nervous system is the most recently understood and highly evolved. The social engagement system has a capacity for self-correcting, complex problem-solving, expressing a large range of emotion, and staying in relationship even in conflict. When motivated by fear, shame, or lack of recognition of our capacity for goodness, we tend to disengage from this evolved system, and default to the older fight, flight, or freeze responses.

Relational

Ethics and power are all about how we treat others by our attitudes and our behavior. Relationships are what make ethics necessary. In a conversation, a colleague challenged: "This isn't an ethics course, this is 'Relationship 101'." Being sensitive to our impact and staying connected even in conflict is, however, the core of ethical relationships. Relationships are most effective and grievances are avoided when we are able to resolve problems and repair connections.

Heartful

Right use of power is the heart of ethics. Empathy and compassion can inform often complex and challenging situations, so that both caregivers and clients will be empowered to self-correct and grow into more sensitivity. The development of compassion, "as being an ability to imagine [and feel] the connection between everyone and everything, everywhere"[vi] is the salve for wounds and separation, and the inspiration and motivation for those who are in positions of power and trust. We can source our power with heart.

Reparational

We all make mistakes. Our impact is often different than our intention. We carry projections from past hurts and wounds. There are difficulties that arise in the course of care giving relationships. Often, we automatically and habitually link present conflict with past trauma. When conflict triggers old trauma, we may disengage from relationships, dissociate, lose touch with our resources, and/or blame others. By approaching ethics and power reparationally, we can put our attention toward skillful resolution, relationship repair, and self-correction. This viewpoint supports engaging in discussion about ethical issues and concerns with colleagues, and attending to conflicts <u>within</u> the relationship instead of feeling ashamed, accused, or out of touch with our impact on others.

Pro-active

Responses to issues of power and ethics can be unconscious and history-based, littered with automatic behavior and outdated beliefs. By actively exploring our ethical edges, taking care of ourselves, asking for and using feedback constructively, we become more sensitive. We can increase our skills, change ineffective habits, and use learnings from our history to grow. Focusing on pro-active right use of power takes ethics to a deeply refined level.

Experiential

Having a felt sense of the impact of the power differential is the key to understanding professional ethical issues. Experiential study using the full spectrum of experiential channels is the most effective method of learning. Studies show that we remember 90% of what we say and do, compared to 10% of what we read.[vii] Ethics, power dynamics, and compassion are best embodied through personal, practical, and engaging experience.

The Vision for Right Use of Power

Power is the capacity to initiate change. Influence is the realized potential for change. The spiraling journey to mastery in the use of power and influence is numinous and potent. Use of personal and role power in a self-led way is both a right and a responsibility.

Those who learn to use their power consciously, caringly, and skillfully are familiar with their profession's code of ethics and with contemporary ethical issues. They have done personal work with their power history and beliefs. They are centered in their ethical compass, are willing to be held responsible for their behavior and can self-correct. They know how to track for and resolve difficulties whenever possible within the therapeutic relationship. They have proactively self-assessed for their "ethical edges," understand dynamics around power, and are actively engaged in the empowered and empowering use of power. They are no longer power-blind.

Four Aspects of Right Use of Power and Influence

In the Power Spiral model, there are four aspects: it is informed, compassionate, connected, and skillful. In the book, sets of informational material are grouped with each of these components, and organized around a circular map of the four cardinal, seasonal, and elemental directions.

Throughout the book, you will find additional names that describe each dimension. Below is a visual map to guide your way around the spiral beginning at #1 *(right hand side, east direction, then moving clockwise.)*

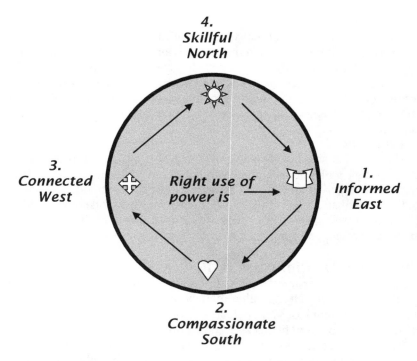

4.
Skillful
North

3.
Connected
West

Right use of
power is

1.
Informed
East

2.
Compassionate
South

Inspirations for the Navigational and Process Maps: A personal story

After returning from my second trip to a remote Outback Station in Arnhemland, Australia, I had a potent dream. I was writing a book, a very unusual book as it was written and was to be read from the inside out, like a spiral. It was quite visual, with pictures and designs that linked from one part of the book to another. I thought the book was supposed to be about my experiences with the Aboriginal people whom I came to love. The title in the dream was to be, "Lessons and Blessings from the Black Soil Country." The title was a mystery to me because the Aboriginals think of their land as the red soil land. In working with the Right Use of Power, I have had the insight that the design for the book, and the spiral process of becoming more skillful, sensitive, and compassionate in using power, is the concept that the dream foretold.

Like my dream, the program is organized in a series of spirals that nest together like rings on a bulls-eye, that radiate outward like the ripples from a stone dropped in a clear pond, that accordion in and out like a slinky. These spirals are organized in resonance with the four cardinal directions of East, South, West, and North. Like the four seasons, each direction has a particular quality—the quality of East is spring, showing up, and new information; South is the quality of Self, awareness, and the burgeoning of growth and color of summer; the West's quality is relatedness and fall harvest and water's flowing connectedness; the quality of North is, like winter, letting go of the leaves of an annual cycle, incubating wisdom, and seeing from a larger perspective. The geographic East of each spiral map is linked to information, South to Self, West to relatedness, and North to wisdom.

I remember asking Audrey, the wise young woman chosen by the Head Man to be the teacher/guide to us "white fellas" what she was going to do about a problematic situation with one of the children. She thought for a long time and then picked up a stick and started drawing a circle in the dirt describing the aspects of her processing of what to do as she went around the circle. "If this happens, then..." A decision came out of moving around the circle attending to the information coming into the circle from the land on all sides. Like Audrey's cycling process, there are a number of such circular processes for working with issues in this program. The answer is often not found in a straight line.

We white fellas had a linear day by day plan for our time in the Outback. In our agenda, it was the day to learn about how didjeridoos are made. When we mentioned this, Audrey looked at us as if we were kindergarteners and said, 'You know, we can go look for didjeridoo trees, but we aren't going to find any, because today isn't a didjeridoo day." We went looking, and Audrey was right, putting our ears to the trees and giving a shake, we didn't hear the sound that indicates a tree is ready to become a didjeridoo.

Similarly, as you absorb the material here, sometimes you will want to "take your seat" in the center of the power spiral and notice where you need to turn next: toward information, or skillfulness, or relatedness, or compassionate awareness. At other times, you will find that by beginning in the east and moving clockwise, gathering information leads to deeper awareness; which leads to more caring and connectedness; which then leads to increased wisdom and skill; which leads to more information and so on.

With the Aboriginal people questions were never answered immediately as we often do in the West. A question was something to be lived with, pondered, forgotten and found again. One day a question was directed to Audrey about the use of some little carved sticks. The question seemed to be ignored and everyone forgot it had been asked. Several days later I realized that Audrey was now giving us the answer. The sticks were used to touch specific points on the head for specific purposes. Audrey said, "This place puts a baby to sleep." Likewise, she described the meaning for many other spots. Ethical concerns and issues of power often don't have immediate, clear, obvious, documented answers. We sometimes need to listen, make space, and gather information from a number of sources.

Other inspirations: Lessons and Blessings

There are other sources of creativity and guidance that have influenced the development of the Right Use of Power approach.

In a group leadership training ten years ago, David Patterson and Amina Knowlan[viii] referred to ethics as "the right use of power and influence." My associations with ethics had been quite dry, formal and imposed. I had felt nervous about acting unethically, even though I knew I didn't want to cause any harm. In a moment of relief and excitement, I saw that ethics as right use of power was an idea I could engage with. It was an idea that had heart. This concept began to transform ethics from a list of unethical behaviors to ethics as relational and compassionate. It inspired me to want to learn more about my power and its impact on others. It gave me the idea I could be both powerful and heartful. This was ethics that could be learned from the inside out instead of from the outside in.

Power has been a life-long personal and professional theme. Through years of ceremonial dancing and personal and spiritual work, my community, Earth Song, worked with and learned from the four directions, with qualities as described in the navigation and process maps. We used a model developed by Elizabeth Cogburn.[ix] We also used Angeles Arrien's "Four Fold Way,"[x] (see Dimension Four Overview) and Ron Kurtz's Sensitivity Cycle[xi] (see Challenges chapter). These became the Four Dimensions of the Power Spiral. Each dimension is a unit of material with a particular focus and each includes and builds on the previous dimension. Collaboratively, we learned about the dynamics of leading and following. We practiced honoring instead of denying our power and had more and more moments of using it with magnificence.

The Hakomi Method of Body-Centered Psychotherapy has been my professional foundation since 1980. The Hakomi Method is the essence of power with heart. The core of the method is the integrated use of mindfulness, the body, and non-violence in psychotherapy. Hakomi has influenced this ethics approach in more ways than I can name. One way is the focus on mindful self-study. My experience is that experiential teaching creates a dynamic atmosphere for personal engagement, excitement, and powerful, life-changing learning. Hakomi inspires my determination to teach and support professional compassion and empowerment--standing in strength and coming from the heart.

Right Use of Power and Influence can be learned.

Right use of power and influence can be learned. This learning happens through a spiraling process of gaining understanding and skillfulness at higher and higher levels of complexity, inclusivity, and transcendence. In fact, right use of power and influence must be learned because good intentions and obeying ethics codes, while essential, are not enough because of a number of factors that are explored in this book:

Factors that make good intentions not enough for right use of power at the highest levels.

* power-blindness....page 3, 5
* impact of the power differential....page 35 plus
* cognitive strategies....page 90
* shame....page 115 plus
* flight/fight/freeze responses....page 117
* non-ordinary states....page 129 plus
* transference....page 155 plus
* difference between intention and impact....page 167 plus
* not enough time and/or support....page 179 plus
* inadequate self-care, stress, burn-out...page 251 plus
* unskillfulness....pages 245-248, 297-300,
* cultural or contextual differences....pages 269-271
* unconscious beliefs that interfere....pages 300-303
* negative effects of elevated role power....pages 304-307
* power paradox....pages 316-319

Summary of the Dimensions

On the next two pages, you will find a concise summary of the material covered in each dimension of the power spiral.

Dimension One: Guided Use of Power • *Own your role power and track your influence.* • *Use your ethical guidelines and moral compass.* • *Work with the dynamics created by the power differential.* Focus on INFORMATION	**BE INFORMED AND PRESENT** This dimension is about **guidance** of many kinds: • owning and having a felt sense of the impact of the power differential role (its potential, its responsibilities, its distortions, and its vulnerability for those in down-power roles) as the basis for all ethical guidelines; • understanding and being guided by information contained in ethical codes as they are wisdom culled from the lived history of our professions; • tracking your impact, and gathering and effectively using information from clients and students; • paying attention to inner guidance and humanistic and spiritual values; • making informed ethical decisions in complex or challenging circumstances and in everyday attitudes and interactions;
Dimension Two: Conscious Use of Power • *Understand & use your history well.* • *Stay present and engage your curiosity.* • *Infuse your power with heart.* Focus on SELF-AWARENESS	**BE COMPASSIONATE AND AWARE** This dimension is about **Self-awareness**: • understanding and learning from your attitudes, beliefs, wounds, and habits in relation to issues of power and authority; • engaging curiosity about yourself and your clients as a deepening and safety-enhancing skill and attitude; • showing up and staying attentive • standing in your strength while staying in your heart. • exploring your empowered and disempowered selves and how your use of power and influence effects others; • working with shame as a power issue because it isolates and de-resources; • practicing compassion as a resonating concern for all.

Dimension Three: **Responsible Use of Power** • *Use the 150% principle.* • *Track your impact and stay connected.* • *Resolve and repair.* **Focus on** **RELATIONSHIP**	**BE CONNECTED AND ACCOUNTABLE** In this dimension the focus is on **relationship**: • increasing skillfulness in tracking for difficulties and staying current in care-giving relationships; • recognizing that your impact is often different from your intention; • being guided by the 150% principle of greater responsibility held by the person in the up-power role; • recognizing that we all make mistakes; understanding how relationship difficulties, when either ignored or dismissed, can escalate to grievance processes; • practicing staying connected even in conflict and using conflict to clarify and resolve difficulties; • attending to relationship repair and using apology effectively.
Dimension Four: **Wise Use of Power** • *Be proactive with yourself and others.* • *Ask for and use feedback well.* • *Self-reflect, self-correct and let go.* **Focus on** **SKILL**	**BE SKILLFUL AND PROACTIVE** This dimension is about cultivating **wisdom**: • understanding that doing the right thing is more effective when it's done wisely; • deepening skill in identifying tendencies, beliefs, and barriers that may make you vulnerable to specific misuses of power; • understanding good self-care as vital for wise use of power; • reflecting on examples of misuses of professional power and learning about the shadow aspects of increased power; • practicing sensitive and skillful down-power influence; • practicing and refining the skills of asking for, receiving, giving, and using feedback; • becoming more skillful at knowing when and how to persist and when and how to let go; • being nourished by wise and skillful uses of power as a social force for good.

Topic Chart

What follows is a visual chart of the topics that are linked to each dimension of the power spiral in this book.

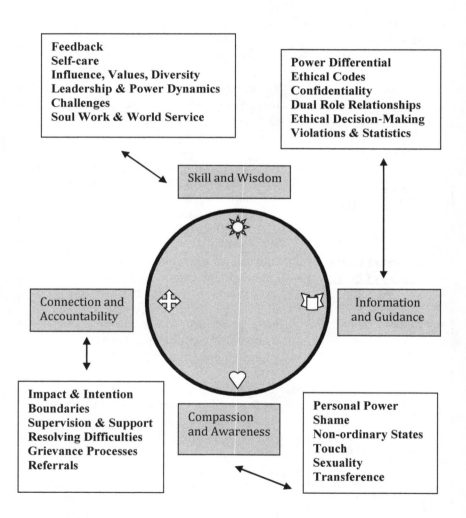

Feedback
Self-care
Influence, Values, Diversity
Leadership & Power Dynamics
Challenges
Soul Work & World Service

Power Differential
Ethical Codes
Confidentiality
Dual Role Relationships
Ethical Decision-Making
Violations & Statistics

Skill and Wisdom

Connection and Accountability

Information and Guidance

Impact & Intention
Boundaries
Supervision & Support
Resolving Difficulties
Grievance Processes
Referrals

Compassion and Awareness

Personal Power
Shame
Non-ordinary States
Touch
Sexuality
Transference

Power Spiral

The Power Spiral is a spiraling guide for increasing sensitivity and consciousness of ethical awareness in everyday practice. You can think of spirals as moving up, down, in toward the center, or expanding outward. Spirals are involved in circular movement, returning to a similar, but different place each time around. Spirals and cycles are models for the natural process of growth. Certainly, the seasons and DNA helix reflect this model. Remember "slinkies," those toys made of tightly-coiled wire? Slinkies are flexible. Not too serious, they propel themselves down stairs on their own. When stretched out you can see and touch each individual spiral ring, and when collapsed they make one solid whole ring. Each of the dimensions of ethical awareness is also its own four directional circle. As a diagram:

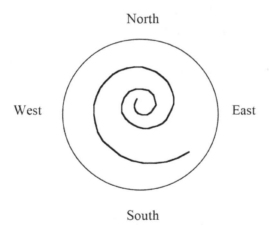

The power spiral is made up of many circular maps. Linking them together creates a spiral. The Power Spiral serves both as a map of the territory of ethics and power issues, and as an acknowledgement that the learning process is a spiral of increasing depth and complexity. Ken Wilber[xii] describes development as "a wonderfully organic, streaming, and spiraling affair." Learning is less linear and more like an ascending spiral toward mastery, punctuated by moments of fresh new awareness and skill. It is more a gestalt than a line.

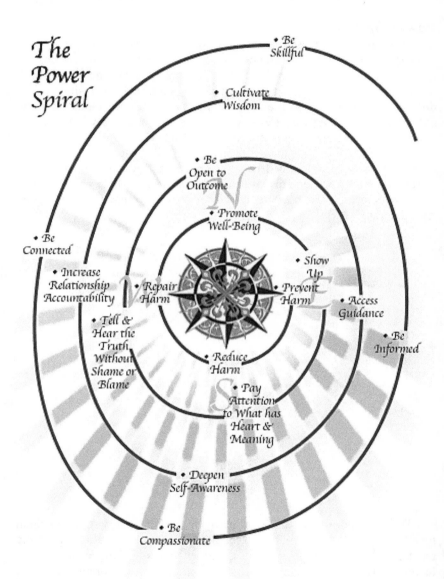

The
Power
Spiral

• Be
Skillful

• Cultivate
Wisdom

• Be
Open to
Outcome

• Promote
Well-Being

• Be
Connected

• Show
Up

• Increase
Relationship
Accountability

• Repair
Harm

• Prevent
Harm

• Access
Guidance

• Tell &
Hear the
Truth
Without
Shame or
Blame

• Be
Informed

• Reduce
Harm

• Pay
Attention
to What has
Heart &
Meaning

• Deepen
Self-Awareness

• Be
Compassionate

Real learning gets to the heart of what it means to be human. Through learning we recreate ourselves. Through learning we become able to do something we never were able to do. Through learning we re-perceive the world and our relationship to it. Through learning we extend our capacity to create, to be part of the generative process of life. There is within each of us a deep hunger for this type of learning. Peter Senge[xiii]

Working with the Power Spiral is a feedback loop. You give to it. It gives to you. You may work with the spiral by moving around it clockwise. You may work with it from the center, receiving at each aspect information from a different vantage point. You may approach the Power Spiral by starting exactly where you are. For example, you might be well-informed about behavioral ethical codes, but need more awareness about the impact of your personal history with power woundings, so you may enter through the aspect of awareness. Or, you may have enough

Core of Right Use of Power

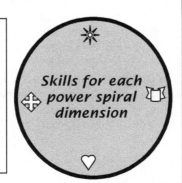

- *Be proactive with yourself and others*
- *Ask for and use feedback*
- *Self-reflect, correct and let go*

- *Use the 150% principle*
- *Track your impact and stay in right relationship*
- *Resolve and repair*

Skills for each power spiral dimension

- *Own your role power & track your influence*
- *Use your ethical guidelines & moral compass*
- *Work with the dynamics created by*

- *Engage your curiosity and use your history well*
- *Stay present and receptive*
- *Infuse your power with heart*

awareness, but be so crippled by shame that you have difficulty being accountable and thus approach the spiral through the relationship aspect in the West. You may be caring and accountable, but naive about power dynamics and need to acquire more skillfulness and so would enter through the North.   Each dimension has three skills and wisdoms.

Power and Heart

Power is the ability to have an effect. It could also be considered the ability to access and mobilize resources. Combining this strength with deep compassion in the spiraling journey to mastery is numinous and potent. It brings together personal development and soul work (being) with creation and accomplishment (doing). Love and creativity yearn to be expressed in form. Being resourced by both personal and role power in the full use of Self is a right and a responsibility.

Much is accomplished when we can embrace and use our personal and professional power with heart and are actively engaged in the right use of this power for the good of all. Becoming familiar with our profession's code of ethics and with contemporary ethical issues combined with doing personal work with our power history and beliefs, we become more skillful in staying related through conflict and keeping our relationships repaired.

We are willing to be held responsible for our behavior. We can self-correct. We have proactively self-assessed for our ethical edges, and understand key dynamics around power,

Spiral by spiral we can reach out our hands, not to strike or defend, but to compassionately relate. Our power and influence will be felt as peace and mutual well-being. This ethic synergizes power with the resonating concern of compassion. The formula is simple and yet mastery is a lifetime practice. Right Use of Power is power with heart, activated from the inside out. Be informed, Be compassionate, Be related, Be skillful.

As caregivers, we are in a powerful position to be influential leaders in the evocation and evolution of an ethic of power and heart. A revolution in ethics and spirit is no longer waiting in the wings.

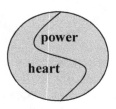

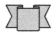

Dimension One: Be Informed

Topics covered in this section:
Power Differential
Codes & Guidelines
Confidentiality
Dual Role Relationships
Ethical Decision-Making
Violations & Statistics

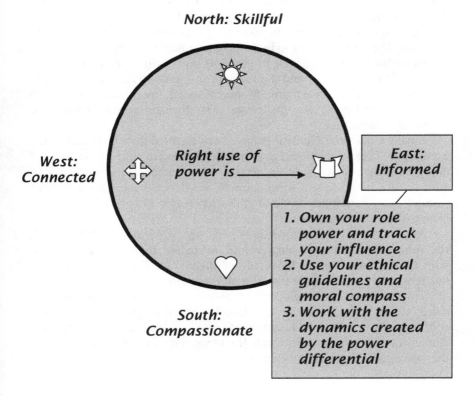

North: Skillful

West:
Connected

Right use of
power is ⟶

East:
Informed

1. *Own your role power and track your influence*
2. *Use your ethical guidelines and moral compass*
3. *Work with the dynamics created by the power differential*

South:
Compassionate

Focus on Information
- *Right Use of Power is Informed*
- *Dimension One is about Guidance:*
  - *Cultivating a felt sense of the impact of the power differential*
  - *Understanding ethical behavior as prescribed in ethical codes and guidelines*
  - *Gathering information from your clients about their experience, needs, and preferences*
  - *Paying attention to and using your values and your inner guidance and sensitivity*

Power Spiral Topics—Guidance Section
The diagram on the previous page is a four directional model. This four directional model is inspired by the qualities of the four seasons and the sacred tree,[xiv] the Sensitivity Cycle from Ron Kurtz, the Four-Fold Way by Angeles Arrien, and the New Song ceremonial dance of Elizabeth Cogburn. These are referred to in the opening chapter on Power and Heart.

Note that the informed use of power is on the right side of the power spiral. This is in the East and the focus is on information. The three skills and wisdoms in the East are: to be informed, own your power and influence, and know your guidelines. The topical material covers the following information.

Ethical Codes and Guidelines have been distilled through accumulated experience. These guidelines have been determined to support the value of doing no harm and acting in the service of our clients. Reading a code of ethics is like listening to a wisdom circle of elders sharing what they have learned. Each item in any code of ethics represents what has been learned from a history of mistakes.

At the core of ethical codes is the concept of the **power differential, the inherently increased power and influence that caregivers have with their clients simply by virtue of their role.** The strong impact of this power differential is the basis for all professional ethics codes.

This section includes guidelines common to most codes. In addition, since Codes of Ethics are continually evolving, topics concerning confidentiality, dual role relationships, use of internet technology (in Dimension, and therapeutic touch (in Dimension 2), are included since they are issues of particular complexity.

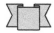

Shame, guilt, fear, and paranoia are often associated with ethics violations. Included in this section are some actual statistics and examples of behaviors that have been grieved. These are presented in order to convey the realities of the small percentage of practitioners who are grieved and the wide range of situations and behaviors covered by complaints.

Caregivers are involved in ethical decision-making in the everyday aspects of client care through the attitudes and manner in which they relate to clients, as well as how they respond to the rarer, and often urgent, ethical challenges and dilemmas. A four step process for ethical decision-making is included in this section.

All of us need to know and understand our profession's ethical guidelines. In addition, in the Right Use of Power approach, being informed also includes accessing and using other kinds of information, e.g.: seeking and paying attention to what your clients tell you, through words or body information, about who they are, what they need, and how they are relating to you. We learn here to pay attention to information that we get through our own perceptions and guidance systems. Gathering information from other resources may also be needed and may include: colleagues, supervision, books, internet, spiritual practices, and internal resources.

Three Skills and Wisdoms

- *Own your role power and influence.*

  You **do** have increased power and influence in your professional role. When you own this increase and understand the dynamics of this role power, you can use it to support and empower your clients.

- *Use your ethical guidelines and your moral compass.*

  Ethical codes are rich sources of history and support. Take time to get to know them. Stay in touch with your integrity, values, and moral center. Access and use all the information that is relevant and available to you. This includes information from codes, research, supervision, your education and experience, your clients and yourself.

- *Work with the dynamics created by the power differential.*

  The increased power brings responsibilities, potential for healing and growth, distortions, vulnerability and shadow aspects. Track the behavioral and cognitive effects on people in both up- and down-power roles.

Barriers and Resources to Information

One aspect of becoming more proactive in the use of our personal and role power is to discover and work with unconscious "Barriers." We may have to increase our wisdom and skill in each dimension. Refer to the Challenges chapter in Dimension Four.

These include **barriers** to understanding ethical information that are habits that interfere with our ability to gather, understand, and use information about ethics. Some of the common barrier habits include getting continually confused, choosing not to read the code at all, or dismissing or disregarding the information. These habits are held in place by beliefs such as, "I'm a good person, therefore I won't cause any harm." "I don't need rules. I'll use my common sense." "If I find out about the guidelines, I might discover I've done something wrong." "I just don't understand what all this emphasis on ethics is all about." "I already know all these things." Personal understanding about the above habits and beliefs is freeing and enlightening.

After personal exploration in this section, participants have said, "I don't want to abuse my power by under-using it ever again." "I want to now actively nourish the right use of my power." "I now understand how and why I stop myself from knowing and the reason is fear." "Thinking of ethics codes as lived wisdom is inspiring. I see them in a different way now."

There are **Resources** in each dimension as well as Barriers. The resources that support the Informed use of power include your profession's Ethical Code, your skillfulness in tracking, understanding, and responding to a broad range of information, and your resourcefulness to consult others as needed.

Power Spiral Layer—Dimension One

The power spiral, like a layer cake, or better yet, a slinky, has multiple layers or spirals. The layer associated with the East dimension is the layer that describes four aspects of the Right Use of Power. The primary edict: "Do no harm" expands to larger purpose and meaning. Right Use of Power affirms the use of personal and role power to prevent harm, and in addition, to reduce harm, repair harm, and promote experiential and sustainable well-being for all. As you can see in the diagram, the first dimension focuses on using power to prevent harm by owning your power and knowing your guidelines. Moving around the spiral, the topics in each dimension relate to the uses of power as named here.

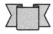

**Promote Well-being
and the Common Good**

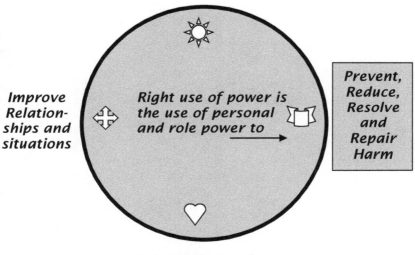

**Prevent,
Reduce,
Resolve
and
Repair
Harm**

**Improve
Relation-
ships and
situations**

*Right use of power is
the use of personal
and role power to*

**Balance Strength
with Compassion**

Ethics is dry without the heart and wisdom which expands ethics from a moral code of behavior to a way of showing love, becoming a better person, family member and health care provider. In this way it enhances servicing and doing world work in the real sense of everyday relationships. I like how you've presented this in your book.

Kamala Quale

Ethics is the ongoing process of applying principles of higher intelligence to the problems of personal and collective existence, and endowing life with values that support the well-being of all. Ethics is the care we show in effecting the lives of others as well as a sense for where one's greatest value lies in relation to others. Ethics might be summarized as cause and effect in balance and applied for the greatest good.

Glenda Green

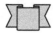

Power Differential

"I'm trying to imagine ethics without an awareness of power. That would be like trying not to step on anyone's toes, without an awareness of one's feet."[xv]

The power differential is the inherently greater power and influence that helping professionals have as compared to their clients. Understanding both the value and the many impacts of the power differential is the core of ethical awareness. Written codes for ethical behavior are based on the strong positive and negative impacts of this power differential.

Clients are in a position in which they must trust in the knowledge and guidance of their caregiver. This difference results in a greater than ordinary vulnerability on the part of the client. Consequently, clients are unusually susceptible to harm and confusion through misuses (either under- or over- use) of power and influence.

"The impact of the role, control, and power difference between client and therapist is very strong and also very subtle, and thus demands a strong ethical stance. In brief, your role as the therapist [or any helping professional] is to create a safe space, empower your client, protect your client's spirit, and to see a wider perspective."[xvi]

Stated in another way, there is a power inequality whenever you take on a role that gives you authority over another or creates the perception that you have that authority. Power differential roles include:

Supervisor	Clergy
Body worker	Healer
Lawyer	Coach
Group leader	Therapist
Counselor	Doctor/Nurse
Mediator	Teacher
Social Worker	Massage Therapist
Guide	Social Worker

Two kinds of power: personal power and role power

In talking about the power differential, it is necessary to clearly describe and distinguish between three kinds of power. This distinction is important because it makes clear that the increased power that accompanies a position of authority is role-based and not the same as personal power.

• Personal power is our birthright ability to have an effect and to have influence.

• Role power is the add-on additional power (and responsibility and opportunity) that accompanies a positional role.

I like to show the difference between these two powers with scarves. When I am a therapist, I have my personal power, of course, but I wear my added-on role power as if it were a scarf around my shoulders. When I leave my office, I take my role-power scarf off. My personal power stays with me. It's like my scarf has access to and stores information related to the enhanced power that belongs to my role. With my scarf on, I can remember multiple details about my client's process. When I take my scarf off, I can and need to leave those details and responsibilities behind. This is not a completely black and white thing. Of course, I continue to have concern about my clients, and I am known as a therapist or teacher even when I am not in these roles. But many misuses of power are a result of the person in the up-power role over-identifying with their role power, forgetting that this is a role-based add-on power. *Story: My friend Nancy's husband is a commercial airline pilot. Until they understood this dynamic, their marital relationship was quite compromised each time Daniel came home and acted as if he were still the airline pilot--a commanding position. Things changed when Daniel ritually took off his hat with the symbolic words, "I'm hanging the pilot on the hook now."*

Third kind of power: status power

I want to name a third kind of power. In contrast to personal power and role power, status power is unearned power though it has some similarities to role power. Status power is much more complex and shifting and has negative impacts that are particularly difficult for the up-status person to understand and respond to. Having increased power through status is like putting on any number of scarves that are visible to down-status people and generally invisible to up-status people. There is further discussion of status power and its relationship to racism, violence and discrimination in the section on *Rankism* on page 33 and in the *Influence, Values, Diversity* chapter, pages 274-277. Please understand that status power is outside the main focus of this book about the ethics of personal and role power.

Here is a chart that summarizes these kinds of power.

PERSONAL POWER (PP)	ROLE POWER (RP)	STATUS POWER (SP)
• PP is our birthright. It is our individual ability to have an effect or to have influence. • It is accompanied by the inherent human right to be treated with dignity, respect, and fairness. • Although PP is always present, we can be more or less aware of it and have more or less access to it. • Our PP can be limited by ourselves and by the misuse of power by others, but in most situations, we can retain some PP through positive attitudes and self-respect. • We can learn to use our PP better in both up-power and down-power roles. • PP comes in many forms, including the power of communication (articulateness), presence (charisma), and creativity. • Can be developed.	• RP, or Positional Power, is earned, awarded, elected or assigned. It is a power add-on. • RP is separate from our PP and is thus mutable. It automatically accompanies any position of authority. • RP carries an increased or expanded amount of power and responsibility. • It is integrated with PP. SP often accompanies RP. • Up- and down-power dynamics create the need for ethical guidelines since those who are down-power are more vulnerable and at risk of harm. • Some assigned roles carry greater increased power and responsibility than others and thus will have a greater negative or positive impact on others. Examples: Doctor/Nurse Teacher/Principal Coach Employer Clergy Chairperson Therapist/Social worker Elected Official Chief Executive Officer Supervisor Parent (special situation) Director Bodyworker Police Officer	• SP is enhanced personal power and influence that is culturally conferred. • SP brings unearned privileges and opportunities. It confers responsibilities, dynamics, and influence that often go unrecognized. • Those with high SP are often unaware of having it. The fish, according to the saying, are the last to know they are in water. Higher status is used to justify racism, violence, and discrimination. • SP depends on cultural values. Thus it may change from culture to culture. Examples: Age Wealth, Celebrity Race Sexual Orientation Nationality Gender Physical Appearance Social Class Physical Prowess Religious Affiliation

Two kinds of roles: up-power and down-power

I refer to those in positions of increased role power as having "up-power" and those in the corresponding positions of lesser power and having "down-power." These are simple and directional terms not intended to indicate disrespect, disempowerment, exploitation or manipulation, better or worse, or power over or power under. Instead, these terms are intended to denote role differences in responsibility and in vulnerability.

Up-power and down-power positions have cognitive, emotional and somatic differences. As an exercise, I ask my students to walk around the room imagining walking with someone up-power to them. My students notice a variety of things--feeling smaller, more cautious, protective, turned inward (or, for some, feeling relaxed, eager, relieved). Then when imagining walking with someone they are up-power with, they notice feeling more spacious, focused on the other, taller, kind and caring, alert. It is very clear to them that the two roles are experienced differently. For most, this is a surprise. A student described the difference in this way: *"When I'm a practitioner, my personal needs and 'stuff' are behind me resting against my shoulders, and when I'm a client, my personal needs and 'stuff' are sitting right there in a huge ball on my lap, visible and available."*

We move back and forth daily between being in up-power positions and down-power positions. *(Like putting on a scarf or robe when in role and taking it off when leaving the role, we move from up-power therapists to a down-power supervisee, or up-power doctor to down-power patient, for example.)* We are usually unaware of the shift. This unconscious shifting of roles makes it more difficult to clearly understand the dynamics and impacts.

Some up-power roles carry a stronger differential than others and therefore a stronger risk of harm, than others. For example, the President of the World Bank or a Policeman or a Therapist have greater power difference than the Chair of a Committee or a Clerk in a store. But all up-power roles have impacts and dynamics.

Value of the Power Differential

In the helping professions, the power differential has great value. Used wisely and appropriately, it creates a safe, well-boundaried, professional context for growth and healing. More specifically, when used ethically and effectively, the power differential offers clients, students, supervisees, and patients some very important assurances.

- Confidence in their caregiver's knowledge, training and expertise
- Security, safety and protection
- Role boundary clarification and maintenance
- Assessments of progress
- Sensitivity, respect, fairness and care
- Allocated responsibilities
- Provision of direction, focus, treatment, guidance, support
- Over view and access to a bigger picture and wider view of persons and situations
- Chain of accountability
- Facilitated accomplishment of task and purpose
- Final decision-making authority

Or, reducing these values to six categories:

Safety, kindness, and appropriate boundaries
Larger frame
Expertise
Assigned responsibilities
Accountability
Assessment and productivity

Think about it. When you go to a therapist, or doctor, or teacher, you want and need to be in an environment where you can get what you need. You want the environment to be different than just talking to a friend. Beyond therapy, when you get on a plane you want and need the pilot to look and act competent. Wearing jeans and a t-shirt just wouldn't do. You need him or her to be skilled, embrace their role and treat you with respect.

Power Differential Responsibilities

There are a number of responsibilities that accompany a power differential role.

- Setting and maintaining appropriate boundaries
- Protecting trust and being trustworthy
- Creating needed safety
- Staying in charge
- Holding the larger container of wholeness and hope
- Being sensitive to your impact
- Inviting and being appropriately responsive to feedback
- Keeping your own personal life in the background so that it won't interfere with being in service to your client

- Tracking and attending to the relationship
- Resolving difficulties and being accountable
- Making an assessment of results
- Keeping appropriate records

Power Differential Opportunities for the Caregiver
This is a good thing! Greater responsibility also means greater opportunity for health and empowerment.
- Healing, preventing and repairing past harm
- Providing a safe relationship and environment
- Promoting well-being and increased empowerment
- Integrating power and heart and offering an experience and model of positive use of power

Understanding and Owning Your Power and Influence
Because the power differential is role dependent, it is easy to over-identify (get inflated or addicted) with this increased or enhanced power. It is just as easy to misuse this increased power by under-identifying with it. The central idea in this first dimension of Right Use of Power is the necessity to understand and own your role power so that you can be conscious and informed. Here are several misunderstandings that illustrate the multiplicity of the impact of the power differential for both helping professionals and clients.

- Believing in equality, you may find it difficult to accept that your role creates a power inequality, and that this inequality is actually essential to your effectiveness.

- Rushed for time, you may underestimate the power differential and over-focus on technique or useful information. Effective use of your role power involves balancing technique with the essential need for relationship connection and repair when needed.

- In fear of manipulative and wounding abuses of power, you may find it difficult to understand that you must own the power that you have, to be able to use it for good. Under-use of power is also a misuse of power.

- Misunderstanding your elevated role power as confirmation of your wisdom and a mandate to take charge, you may inadvertently disempower, disregard, or disrespect your clients.

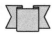

- Motivated by a desire to be of service, you may find it difficult to comprehend that your impact may be different from your intention, and that it may be experienced as confusing or harmful.

Over-use of Role Power

Considerations of the abuse of power typically focus on misuses of power by those in a position of trust that cause harm for clients. Taking advantage of the vulnerability of their clients harms through manipulation, disempowerment, and undue influence. Examples of common grievances or litigations involve taking advantage of or causing harm through sexual contact, providing services outside area of competence, failure to terminate or refer, misrepresenting credentials, and misleading advertising.

Stories: • *An acupuncturist made a diagnosis. His client, being interested in getting as much information as she could, went to another practitioner and was pleased to find that through a very different kind of testing, the diagnosis of the acupuncturist was confirmed. At her next session, she brought him the results. The acupuncturist became very upset and refused to treat this client because she hadn't trusted his diagnosis. Instead of treating her, he spent the session time telling her that for her to be healed she needed to trust him and not try to think things through herself. She then received a bill for the session.*

• The former minister of a church, thinking that he was being supportive and helpful to the new minister, began serving on several committees. He couldn't understand why the new minister felt he was interfering with her leadership. He had overused his power and influence because he didn't recognize that he still had a great deal of influence with members of the church. Understanding and owning role power allows it to be used beneficially.

Under-use of Role Power

Under-use of role power is also a misuse of power. This statement comes as a big "aha" to many caregivers and leaders. Recognizing, valuing, and owning role power and influence is essential to good care. The inherent increased power of a role is not the problem. The problem is when this power is used to put-down, manipulate, shame, or abuse. Caregivers tend to have a force-and-exploitation understanding of power and tend to be oversensitive to abusive and manipulative use of power and thus often dismiss or deny their inherent increased role power. I hear things like, "I refuse to act like I have power over my clients." "I trust my clients to know what is best for them." "I'm very sensitive to issues of diversity and white privilege. I just won't go there. Those words up- and down-power trigger me." "The minute I heard the word down-power, I just collapsed. I never want to cause my clients to feel disempowered by my being up-power." Story: *One of my students, when role-playing being in an up-power role and wearing a scarf to symbolize the additional power of her role, simply took off her scarf and handed it to her partner who was playing the role of client. She didn't want to own her role power. Rather than feeling good about being given the scarf, her client described feeling quite uneasy, even frightened when her partner took off the scarf. She was truly concerned that her therapist would not be capable of providing her with the care and support she needed.* We can treat our clients as equal human beings deserving of respect, and dignity and still value, own and use our role power. Right use of power is learned over a lifetime and calls for skill, awareness, and sensitivity that goes beyond the essential foundation of good intention.

Stories: • *A massage therapist spent most of a session asking her client questions about a debilitating disease, not so that she could treat her better, but to satisfy her curiosity. Her client did not receive an adequate massage. The therapist assumed that her client would tell her if she didn't want to talk about this.*

• *A therapist didn't "take charge" when his client clearly needed strong and specific guidance.*

• *I asked a group of people who run a wonderful program for kids to arrange themselves in the room to represent the hierarchy of power and influence among them. After a chaotic moment all looked toward the founder and director of the group who was moving to the outside edge of the group indicating that she wanted everyone to feel powerful and influential. Someone then said, "You must own your place as the one with most power here. We won't know where to be until you claim your position of power. It's not that we're not powerful. It's paradoxical. We just need a strong center to organize around. When you are direct, we find our places." Then when the director stepped into the center, the whole system became clear.*

Enhanced Effect

Just as power is defined as the ability to have an effect, the power differential can be described as the ability to have an enhanced effect on those in a down-power role. Because of this enhanced impact, hurts or misunderstandings are easily exaggerated. This exaggeration will be even more pronounced with clients who lack personal awareness, are not

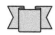

relationally skilled, have low self-esteem, or are impaired by pain or anxiety. These may be the very issues they bring to therapy. Misunderstandings may be experienced as betrayal; touch may be experienced as sexual advance, recommendations may be experienced as demands, and observations may be experienced as criticisms.

Expectations

In an exercise designed to explore the effects of the power differential, half of the participants were asked to stand in the center of the room and the other half to sit in a circle around those in the center.

The seated participants (client position) were asked to imagine themselves as members of a personal growth group and the people in the center (the up-power position) were the leaders of this group. "Notice what expectations you have of your leaders. Understand that some of these expectations may not be very mature or reasonable, just notice and say aloud what they are. And then to the 'up-power people, 'Notice what it's like to hear these'."

Responses included: *"I expect you to care for me unconditionally. I expect you to know what I need even when I don't know. I expect you to be impeccable. I expect you to be trustworthy. I expect you to make it safe for me. I expect you to handle or protect me from other people who are being irritating or mean. I expect you to be 100% fully present. I expect you to understand me. I expect you to hold good boundaries. I expect you not to hurt me."* The clients were surprised at how immature and unrealistic some of their expectations sounded, and that they would not usually have said them aloud; and yet these responses seemed familiar and real. The up-power folks were a bit overwhelmed. "Why would I want to put myself in a position to receive all these expectations! No wonder I feel tense or nervous. I've felt every single one of these." The power differential calls up a lot of usually hidden expectations and projections. Naming them can bring relieving objectivity and the opportunity to differentiate and work with unrealistic expectations directly.

Idealizing and Devaluing

As noted above, clients tend to both idealize and devalue those in the power differential role. In the workshop exercise, the participants in the client role named their idealizations: "You are just amazing! You have changed my life. I wish I had the kind of presence you have. I can't believe you figured that out so quickly. You have healed me." And on the other side, devaluations such as: "You should have known. I can't believe you said that to me. How could you be so insensitive and abrupt. I expected you to live up to your principles. You cut me off. How could you be so wrong."

The idealizing spectrum covers a continuum of expressions that call for different responses. On one end, there are genuine expressions of appreciation, such as "I'm so grateful for your help and support." Receiving and being nourished by these statements is good for the relationship and empowering for your clients. On the other end are the idealized expressions that come from a disempowered place, such as, "You're the best. I wish I had it all together, like you do." These deserve reflective attention: "It's important to you to 'have it all together.' That would be good, huh? Does it interest you to explore this here?"

Empowered appreciation ←—————————→ *Disempowered appreciation*

Likewise, the devaluing spectrum calls for discernment in response. On one side of the spectrum are genuine expressions of difficulty, misunderstanding, or hurt, for example: "I'm don't understand why you said that. I thought you understood me." Attention to the relationship and to relationship repair is what's needed. On the other end of the spectrum are indications of distress that call for attention to and addressing a psychological issue, for example, "You're just like all the others. You just tell me I shouldn't do this and expect it to solve the problem. I'm not a formula."

Relationship difficulty ←—————————→ *Psychological issue*

Over-identification

One of the pitfalls of serving in a role with a power differential has to do with becoming identified with your clients' idealizing or devaluing of you. Then you may become inflated or deflated in response to your clients' opinions.

Story: Alice, a therapist, became so sensitive and defined by whether she was being idealized or devalued, that she had to quit her therapy practice. Without her work, she also found she had lost her identity. She was unable to distinguish between who she was and who her clients thought she was. As she found her way back to the work she loved, she learned to disengage from her client's definitions and to be able to meet the world with more solid and consistent sense of self.

This story illustrates two mistakes you can make. It's a mistake to think a response is **all about you**; and it's a mistake to think that a response is **not at all about you.** Both have the effect of creating a disconnection.

Power Differential, used to promote well-being, is...

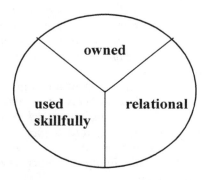

Rankism

In his book *Somebodies and Nobodies,* Robert Fuller[xvii] gives the power differential an even broader meaning in society as a whole. He refers to rank as the seat of power and to the abuse of rank as the root of all forms of discrimination. Rank is our position in any hierarchy, and this rank signals the amount of power we have in the hierarchy—the higher the rank, the greater the power. Ageism, sexism, racism, and anti-Semitism are abuses of rank. Culture, religion, gender, sexual preference, race, socio-economic status, job title, educational level are positions that carry rank with them. Helping professionals by title have a higher rank than clients or office workers. Interestingly, Fuller points out that *"unlike race and gender—native traits that are generally fixed—rank is mutable and in fact is constantly changing. We can hold high rank in one setting (e.g. at home) and simultaneously be low on the totem pole in another (at work)...As a result, most of us have been not only victims but also perpetrators of rankism."* Acknowledging this mutability, helps us engage our sensitivity to any harm caused by misuses of power.

"We [must] understand that it is not race or gender per se that is keeping discrimination alive, but [the] social rank and power we still attach to it. The abuse of the power inherent in rank *"typically takes the form of self-aggrandizement and injurious or discriminatory behavior toward those in positions of lower rank. In some circumstances, the abuse rises to the level of exploitation or oppression".* The misuse of the power differential for helping professionals is rankism. The safety and

effectiveness of the helping relationship is dependent on the right use of the power differential. To reiterate because this is such an important point, *"The trouble is not with rank per se but with the abuse of rank...We rightfully admire and love authorities—parents, teachers, bosses, political leaders—who use the power of their rank in an exemplary way. Accepting their leadership entails no loss of dignity or opportunity by subordinates. In contrast, those who abuse their power by demeaning, exploiting or oppressing those they outrank betray a sacred trust and sow seeds of indignity that ripen into resistance and may ultimately leave their victims thirsting for vengeance."*

As a healing force for the dismantling of all forms of rankism, Fuller proposes a dignitarian society. *"Human beings everywhere have an innate sense that dignity is their birthright and are quick to detect affronts to it...The basic tenet of a dignitarian society is that we are all equal in dignity—not just in theory but in practice, not just in God's eyes but in each others'."* Treating others with dignity is another way of describing the right use of the power differential.

150% Principle

While both parties are responsible for the quality and integrity of the relationship, the practitioner, as the one in the role of greater power, is ultimately responsible for making sure both parties are:

- using their power consciously and skillfully
- being accountable
- resolving a situation when difficulties arise

Those in the client role are
- more vulnerable to misuses of power
- more easily influenced
- more invested in being liked, accepted, and/or respected
- more dependent on and concerned about trust
- have varying abilities to understand and use this role well

Those who are most susceptible to misuses of power
- lack personal awareness
- are not relationally skilled
- are impaired by pain, anxiety, trauma, or shame
- have low self-esteem
- are not clients by choice

I want to highlight two things that are connected to the 150% principle. The 150% principle alludes to the fact that the up-power role is <u>weighted</u> toward responsibilities and the down-power role is <u>weighted</u> toward vulnerabilities. This is the core reason why ethical guidelines are necessary.

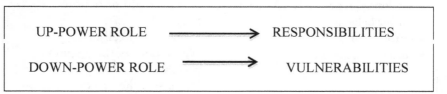

It is also true that those in up-power roles can feel very vulnerable. They sometimes feel afraid, under-confident, overwhelmed, triggered, or compassion-fatigued. And it is true that sometimes those in down-power roles need to take responsibility for changing the system, giving difficult feedback, and being compassionate toward those in authority.

The other is a reminder that in saying yes to the increased power that is embedded in up-power roles, you are also saying a humble yes to receiving guidance, awareness, and information from a source or "field" greater than you. This extra awareness is a gift of the extra 50%.

Summary of Role Differences with their Responsibilities and Liabilities *(Although this book was originally focused toward psychotherapists, this list can be useful to anyone when in a an up-power role or a down-power role.)*

Person in the UP-POWER Role	Person in the DOWN-POWER Role
Is ultimately responsible for the whole or a larger part of the job/project/service. Is in service to clients/students. May take action on down-power person's behalf.	Is responsible for his/her part of the job/project/service. Receives services agreed upon.
Has increased power and influence due to their ability to: • hire/fire/promote and demote • assess: progress/results/	• Has decreased power and is more vulnerable to being rejected, exploited, shamed, taken advantage of, abused, oppressed, disrespected, unduly

effectiveness/performance • prescribe or advise on tasks • deal with problems and people • assign tasks/set standards and expectations • set consequences/reward down-power behavior • enforce rules • make final decisions	influenced, and manipulation than his/her up-power colleagues. • May feel less powerful as a person (not just in his/her role). • May have authority issues triggered. • May have unrealistic expectations of the up-power person. • May assign the up-power person either more or less power than s/he actually has. • May transfer feelings or relationships from the past onto the up-power person.
Must demonstrate trustworthiness and earn trust and not assume that trust goes with the role.	• May either assume or test for trustworthiness.
Role is recognized for expertise, training, or skill. Receives higher pay and greater deference.	Receives lower pay and lesser deference than up-power colleagues.
Sets and maintains appropriate boundaries.	Obeys or challenges boundaries as circumstances dictate.
Has greater influence through his/her words and actions. His/her praise or criticism and respect or disrespect has strong impact.	Can be easily and strongly influenced by the words and actions of up-power persons. This influence can effect his/her dignity and self-esteem.
May have the role-related need to be liked or respected.	Has the role-related need or desire to be liked and respected.
Is expected to provide feedback and direction.	• Risks loss or humiliation by giving challenging feedback,

	asking for change, or being assertive.
Is 150% responsible for good relations and conditions. Note: The 150% Principle describes the extra relationship responsibility born by when in an up-power role.	Is only 100% responsible for good working relationships and conditions and for resolving problems and conflicts.
May be easily idealized and/or devalued.	• May idealize, devalue, and/or have unrealistic expectations of the persons or groups in up-power roles; • Is more likely to escalate conflict when he/she doesn't feel heard or responded to or to withdraw and internalize his/her concerns.
May need to assist client/employee/family member in becoming more empowered, collaborative, respectful, engaged, inspired, confident, appreciated, and/or productive.	• May be disempowered or may unnecessarily disempower him-/herself and become apathetic, disrespectful, angry, unmotivated, disengaged and unproductive. • May need to assist persons in up-power roles to use their power more wisely or skillfully by using down-power influence. • Usually has power to leave down-power position if it is not working well and can't be changed.
May have difficulty understanding the difference and switching between interpersonally focused interactions and task-focused ones but is still 150% responsible for maintaining these two aspects.	May have difficulty understanding the difference and switching between interpersonally focused interactions and task-focused ones.
May imagine or feel all-powerful.	May imagine or feel no power.
May be affected or driven by shadow aspects of power and by faulty justifications for unethical behavior.	May not know what kinds of behavior are unethical.

Some clients experience down-power as no-power. They may give "all" their power to their caregiver; distrust their own knowledge, research, intuition or gut feelings; or be overly self-protective and unrevealing. With these clients, your role opportunity and responsibility is to teach them to be more empowered and engaged in their healing process. You may encourage them to be more collaborative and pro-active. Other clients experience "down-power" in an empowered way. They bring the power of their perceptions, needs, and interests to the care-giving relationship, and take appropriate responsibility for the relationship working well.

It is necessary, however, to remember that even though responsibility is shared, the practitioner is considered to be ultimately more responsible. Marni Harmony,[xviii] a minister, metaphorically calls this the 150% principle—both are 100% responsible and the practitioner is 150% responsible. As a rule, in the most successful helping relationships, the practitioner actively encourages clients to be honest and forthcoming in their responses to the relationship and the services provided. This collaborative feeling reduces the misunderstandings and increases the ease with which difficulties can be repaired. This is what is meant by sharing responsibility for satisfaction and success. However, due to the increased power and influence the person in greater role power, is the one who is 150% responsible for noticing and resolving difficulties and holding established boundaries.

However empowered your clients feel and act, the power differential still has strong impact. A power differential role is different in significant ways from a client role, even for the most aware and experienced clients. "Fish are the last to discover water" is a well-known saying. The powerful may be the last to understand their power. The many and diverse impacts of the power differential are often invisible to those in up-power positions. No shame or blame is intended, but this observation should be strong impetus to make these dynamics visible and understood. Innocent clients may not recognize misuses of the power differential. Aware clients may not be able to successfully address difficulties because of their down-power position. Understanding and supporting role-related empowerment is important and courageous territory for awareness and sensitivity.

Healthy and Harmful Power Spirals

Feedback came in from a student and it was useful and important: *"Yes, now I know the differences between up-power roles and down-power roles. I see that the power differential has its gifts and shadows. But I don't think I understand how the relational dynamics work."* Naming the

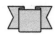

impacts of the power differential is one thing, but knowing how these dynamics can be used to move toward relationship health or harm is another thing. Here are several of the most potent relational dynamics that accompany power differences described in terms of healthy power spirals and harmful power spirals. In a healthy power spiral, the relationship becomes more and more trustworthy, respectful, and collaborative. In a harmful power spiral, the relationship becomes less and less trustworthy, respectful and collaborative. The one in the up-power role has 150% responsibility for the direction the spiral takes.

Here are a number of examples of power differential relationships in which the relationship went into a harmful power spiral. Each story is followed by a suggestion for a "do-over" that could have shifted the situation into a healthy power spiral. There are both one-on-one and group dynamics included. These stories are composites of real situations.

Harmful power spiral story: *James' client came to him upset about some misleading advertising that James had put into a promotional flier. James responded defensively and self-righteously telling his client that it was his marketer who had prepared the flier and so he wasn't responsible. Their therapeutic relationship quickly deteriorated through a series of emails that got more and more accusatory and heated. These emails became pages long and very intense. It was a tragic mess that damaged James' reputation.*

Here's a possible do-over: James could have listened to his client, found out about his feelings, self-reflected and taken responsibility for the flier even though he didn't prepare it, offered an apology and agreed to look over every piece of marketing before it goes out. My guess is that James' client would have been satisfied and gained more trust in James and more confidence that he could offer feedback without getting a lot of defensiveness and push-back. The relationship would have recovered and spiraled upward into more collaboration and health.

What may have interfered with James' ability to get into an upward spiral? Interestingly, after going through this in supervision, James himself was astonished at how confused and off-the-track he'd gotten. Here are his reflections in my words. *"I can't believe how easily my identity as a good, ethical person felt attacked by this comparatively simple feedback. I didn't understand the 150% principle in which I, as the up-power person, am responsible for fliers about me done by my assistant. I am surprised that I felt like it would be weak for me to apologize even after I realized that he was right. I should never, ever have done all this by email. Email leaves a written record that could be used against me and, even more importantly, it distorted the relationship. I caused unnecessary suffering and wasted time and energy."*

Themes: Feedback, 150% principle, apology, internet technology, defensiveness

Harmful power spiral story: *Jude was 35 and owned a yoga studio. He was a good and loved teacher. He and one of his high school age students began having romantic feelings toward each other. They deliberately stayed chaste but planned to be together after she turned 18. They felt like they were in love. The girl's mother and the yoga community suspected they were having an affair and got distressed. After feedback about the concerns got no response from Jude and rumors escalated, the girl's mother reported Jude to the police.*

Possible do-over: Jude had a series of times, as we usually do when we have made a mistake, when he could have turned the situation in a healthy direction. At any point, he could have, with a kind explanation, stopped the romantic relationship. But when he began getting feedback of rumors and concern and feeling the community distress, he could have stopped the relationship and offered an apology to the community. The yoga community could have returned to health.

Here are his reflections in my words: *"I had the idea that this was true love and that love was more important than everything else. I really thought that. So it felt like everyone else didn't understand and were wrong to object. Now I see that I was in a position of authority as the teacher and owner of the studio. This position gave me responsibilities for the little community. Instead, I was prioritizing my own needs and wants. I also didn't understand that teacher/student love usually has a different nature than romantic love between equals. I didn't understand the vulnerability of Sally's situation as a student in my care. I lost everything by not getting that I needed to take care of my responsibilities as owner and teacher. I'm so sorry for my bad choices."*

Themes: prioritizing own needs and desires, 150% principle, feedback, down-power vulnerability, staying connected

Harmful power spiral.

Story: *After several assistants hadn't worked out, Cheryl finally found an assistant, Kay, who was terrific. Cheryl really wanted her to like her job and stay. Almost every week Kay texted wondering if she could shift her work time around. Every time Cheryl re-arranged her scheduled to accommodate. Kay made more requests and Cheryl made more accommodations. Their working relationship was warm and included conversations about their personal lives. Cheryl realized she felt she was being taken advantage of and that tasks were just not getting done. She started avoiding Kay. Kay responded by making more requests. The relationship slipped into a downward spiral.*

Suggested do-over.

This do-over was a conversation initiated by Cheryl that provided a course adjustment. Cheryl realized that she was under-identifying with her up-power role. She wanted Kay to like the job and so she was not being direct about what she needed from Kay as her employee. She was also mixing up friendship and task. To her surprise, after talking honestly about their feelings, Kay was actually relieved to get more direction and guidance and better boundaries. She had been feeling bad about the way that she was ending up making her job less important simply because Kay was so accommodating. Cheryl owned her up-power role and the relationship deepened and the work got done.

Themes: under-identifying with power role, confusing friendship and task, feedback, 150% principle, staying connected, tracking and attending to difficulties right away before they escalate

Harmful power spiral:

Story: *Maya talked about how important feedback was. One of her students, Bob, told her that he was angry about the sloppy time boundaries in the class. A ten-minute break would go on for 30 minutes and Maya, the teacher would often arrive 5 minutes after class was supposed to start. Maya told the student that this was an emergent class and that she had noticed that everyone seemed to be making good use of the time that they had to wait for her that morning. She asked Bob, since time boundaries were so important to him, to take leadership of the time. When he called people back after a stated 10-minute break, Maya told him that, as the leader of this group, it didn't work well because she was so busy during break that she didn't have time to get a snack. No surprise that the class fell apart and things got worse.*

Suggested Do-over:

Maya could have listened to Bob's feelings, gotten curious about how others in the group felt, and depending on group consensus, tried an experiment with more accurately assessing the time needed for break. She could have apologized for arriving late and not sticking to the time boundaries she did set, re-acknowledged her up-power responsibility for setting and managing time boundaries, and thanked Bob for bringing this to her attention. This action would have created an upward spiral of increasing trust and engagement.

What got in her way? After a challenging coaching session, these are Maya's reflections. *"Well, lots of these things are painful realizations. I'm so passionate about the potential of emergent design and groups in which everyone comes forth as a leader. I get now that actually I was putting my needs first about timing and imagining that everyone else's needs were similar or would fit in with mine. Big ego, embarrassing. I now understand that starting and ending times are my responsibility. Break times can be flexible, but need to be kept to the stated time or people will be standing around frustrated. That's my job or an assistant's job. Other kinds of leadership can emerge but there are a few responsibilities that are mine. I'm the one being paid. I'm the one with the curriculum. I'm the one attending to safety. And then, because I haven't recognized my up-power role as giving me more power, I didn't realize how risky it was for Bob to speak up. And, after I had said I wanted feedback, I really put him down. Ugh. I guess I just didn't want to give up control and power by apologizing. In retrospect, it would have been so simple to avoid that big blow-up."*

Themes: over-identifying with up-power role, feedback, 150% principle, defensiveness, boundaries, apology

Summary of some attitudes-with-skills-attached to cultivate in working wisely and well with the dynamics set up by a power difference.

• Own your role power	• Self-reflect and self-correct
• Be guided by the 150% principle	• See apology as leadership
• Respond to and use feedback well	• Track, resolve and repair
• Set and maintain good boundaries	• Integrate strength and heart
• Stay present and connected	• Consult often

Alchemy of Yes

> *"Stepping into my power in either role is actually less exhausting."*
> *Serena*

We all know what it's like to be in each role. Therapist and then client, therapist and then supervisee, teacher and then student, assistant and then therapist. Moving from up-power to down-power, down-power to up-power. Usually we are not conscious of this shift. But there are differences that are felt somatically, emotionally, and cognitively. When in down-power role, we are more at risk of being hurt or taken advantage of, receive direction regular assessments, and are much more vulnerable. This position has a "feel" to it. When in up-power mode, we have

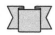

increased power and greater responsibility, we get paid (or paid more), we see the bigger picture, we direct and we make assessments. This position also has a "feel" to it. Saying yes and owning either role takes skill and attention.

Originally, this book was solely focused on helping those in up-power care-giving roles to understand the impacts of the power differential so they could use their up-power roles sensitively and effectively, with less harm and more collaboration. However, over the years I have understood that there are more and less skillful uses of down-power as well. The alchemy of yes results from both partners in the power differential understanding the opportunities embedded in their roles. Here's a little chart to help.

Guidance for Saying Yes when in a Down-power Role	
• showing up and offering your self-awareness	• being willing to give feedback and ask for and suggest a change
• being appropriately cautious and self-protective	• letting go of having to be in charge or in control, yet knowing you have choice
• understanding that the other role--up-power is not ALL power	• understanding that down-power is not NO power and being willing to be appropriately vulnerable and humble
• using down-power influence in sensitive and empowered ways	• knowing that the person in the up-power role, by virtue of the role, will have access to broader or deeper information
• tracking your impact and not taking unnecessary risks; remembering that it is good to do the right thing, but better to do it skillfully	• discerning when to persist and when to let go
	• keeping task responsibilities and friendships separate

Working with some physicians, the exercise was to pair up with one taking the role of doctor and the other the role of patient, while observing their experience. Then they switched roles and imagined being in the other role. When they were in the down-power role, several of these doctors noticed, to their surprise, that it was much more challenging to be in the patient role. They discovered that they were unwilling to shift into the down-power role of being a patient. This meant, in effect, that they were shutting the doctor out and not getting the care and expertise they needed and were paying for.

The quality of relationship, creativity, collaboration and effectiveness that results when both up- and down-power parties say "yes" to their roles is what I call the alchemy of yes. Imagine a group of people standing in two circles with the members of the inner circle facing the members of the outer circle. Those in the inner circle are in an up-power role while those in the outer circle are in a down-power role. In my training, I invite those in the inner circle to think about the ways they say a "half-yes" to their role power. There are many reasons, for example, *"I'm exhausted." "I don't have enough confidence." "I don't like this role." "I didn't choose it." "I'm afraid of causing harm." "I want everyone to like me."* Then they show their "half-yes" in their body and posture. The outer circle in down-power roles experience their responses to their up-power partners. Responses are remarkably dramatic: *"I want to protect myself." "I don't want to engage." "I want to walk away." "My space feels so small." "I don't have confidence that I will get what I need." "I want to take care of her."* Next the up-power people find their "yes" to their role power and embody this "yes." There are striking responses of interest, safety, confidence, spaciousness, willingness and good feeling about the relationship.

We then shift to the outer circle and the down-power people name and embody their "half-yes" to their role. *"I don't trust anyone in authority." "I don't want to give up control." "I'm tired." "I don't want to have to do anything. I just want to be taken care of." "I'm afraid." "Just like always before, this just isn't going to work." "I could be hurt here. Better be very cautious." "I want and deserve to be the leader here."* Up-power participants noticed their responses to their half-yes clients or employees. *"Looks like really hard work to me." "They look so scared underneath the outer shell." "I'm going to have to earn their trust by demonstrating using my power well."* One participant noticed that in her actual job, this is the way most of her clients begin in therapy. In fact, there is wisdom in down-power caution. The down-power role is a high-risk role that requires trust in the good ethics of the up-power person. This trust needs to be earned by demonstrations of personal integrity, and role sensitivity and skill. A down-power participant noted that the more her up-power partner stayed in her "yes," the more he felt better about being in down-power. When the down-power folks found their "yes" to their role, they felt positive, engaged, hopeful, safe and trusting. And when both circles were owning and saying yes to their roles, the relationships felt collaborative and healthy.

Two-sided "yes" relationships are what we strive for and are the most productive ones. Collaborative and healthy relationships are possible and productive within structures that embody a role power difference. Collaboration doesn't require banishing the power differential or making hierarchy the enemy. Hakomi Trainer, Morgan Holford, describes the power differential as *"linear and round at the same time: right use of hierarchy as a vertical linear line and right use of relationship as a circular surround."*

The Alchemy of Yes also reflects the 150% principle: the person in the up-power role still has much greater responsibility for the health of the relationship. In fact, a large part of the up-power role involves earning the trust of the person in the down-power role and helping him or her learn how to make best use of their role.

Summary

The four most potent impacts of the power differential to keep in mind when in an up-power role:

Those in <u>down-power</u> role

1) are more vulnerable and at risk of harm.

2) are only 100% responsible for the health of the relationship while person in up-power role is 150% responsible.

3) take a risk in being direct, and giving negative feedback or suggestions for change.

4) frequently feel or expect to be disempowered,

**Self-study Practice:
Getting a felt sense of the power differential**

---

1. To get a felt sense of this role-related power difference, please set up two chairs: the up-power chair and the down-power chair. As you sit in each chair, settle in to feeling what it is like to be in each role. Note: If you have an actual partner, take turns sitting in each chair. You can imagine and reflect on an up-power role you have (ie. doctor/patient, employer/employee, teacher/student) or you can choose a role you would like to try out (i.e., police officer, king or queen, CEO.)

When in your up-power role, notice your posture, your emotions, and your overall sense of yourself. Then reflect on any or all of the following:

1. Your expectations—of yourself, of the other
2. What is it like to have increased power, responsibility, and opportunity?

3.   What is it like to have training, experience, expertise that you bring to this role?

4.   What is it like to be the one who is paid (or paid more) and receives greater deference?

5.   How do you feel about making assessments about the down-power person's progress and capabilities?

And now move to the other chair, the down-power chair (switch roles if you are with a partner) and mindfully settle into getting a felt sense of yourself in this other role. Notice your posture, emotions, overall sense of yourself

1.   Your expectations—of yourself, of the other
2.   What is it like to have needs--for help, direction, support, or healing?
3.   What is it like to know you will be assessed?
4.   Your level of vulnerability to criticism, rejection, undue influence, disrespect, being taken advantage of?
5.   Will you assume safety and trustworthiness or "test" for it?
6.   What are your hopes? How do you want to be treated?
7.   What are your fears? How could you be hurt?
8.   How are your past experiences effecting you?

Now return to your ordinary consciousness and reflect or draw or write about your experiences in both roles.   Think about how your acknowledgment and sensitivity to this power differential could be translated into your differential role relationships in the future.

2.   Think of a time when you got caught in a harmful power spiral. Using what you now know, how would you do it over?

3.   What are several ways you have in the past said a "half yes" to an up-power role and several ways you have said a "half yes" to a down-power role? What will you do differently now?

A psychotherapists' reflections: *"I have always equated power with power OVER, force, and manipulation. I am now seeing power as a skill, as knowledge, as sensitivity and awareness. This is so different." "I now understand that my clients and I are equals as humans, but we have different roles. These roles have significant differences." "The new paradigm of power requires the therapist to educate their clients about their use of power."*

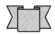

Ethical Codes & Guidelines

"All good people who have power over others, even just a little power and even for just a little while, need access to an ethic that can guide their use of it." — *Perry London[xix]*

Many caregivers, when asked to name their spontaneous associations with ethics and ethical codes, respond with gratitude, appreciation, and interest. However, many others have responses similar to the following.

"Oh, I already know about ethics. There are three rules: 1) don't sleep with your clients, 2) don't sleep with your clients, 3) don't sleep with your clients." • *"I feel, let's see, upright when I think about ethics."* • *"Ethics is so, well, stuffy."* • *"Ethics is like a dirty word. You read about it and then you don't talk about it."* • *"I want to be good. I don't need to be scared into it."* • *"I just feel myself getting tenser and more paranoid whenever I read through the code. It seems so self-righteous, strict, and complex. Some of the details are so ridiculously fussy."* • *"I get an image of a beautiful piece of lace—so very intricate, and yet so 'straight-laced.'"* • *"I can barely stay connected while I read, and I just want to 'space out' and pray that none of it happens to me."* • *"I experience such a disconnect between what we say and what we do."* • *"It's a legalistic and punitive system that I don't want anything to do with."*

An ethical code is a document of accumulated experience describing behaviors that have been determined to cause or potentially cause harm. Over the past few years, ethical codes are increasingly written in positive form to describe behaviors that protect clients from harm. Having the felt sense of the power differential as you experienced it in the self-study practice in this program provides the foundation for understanding the reasoning behind the behaviors prescribed in ethical codes and guidelines. Ethical codes are not arbitrary rules or regulations. Understanding a code of ethics is similar to listening to a wisdom circle of elders sharing what they have learned. Each item in a code represents something that has been learned from a history of mistakes.

The value of ethical codes and guidelines

- To benefit from the lived wisdom of healers, teachers, and caregivers. This wisdom contains knowledge of specific behaviors that can cause harm to clients.

- To provide easily accessible and specific behavioral guidance to practitioners who are facing ethical dilemmas.

- To publish and make available common professional standards that our clients can count on and know are in their best interests.

- To offer a "standard of care," grounded in a set of consistent and specific behaviors and attitudes.

- To increase awareness of areas of possible harm that may not be obvious.

- To provide a set of guidelines to which caregivers formally agree to be held accountable.

- To honor the potency of transference and counter-transference.

Challenges

There are also some challenges associated with ethical codes. The responses of the students quoted at the beginning of this chapter describe the first challenge: ethical codes are often experienced as excessively detailed, formal and imposed, unattainable and rigid. For some, following the ethical rules seems to promote relationships with clients that are technically proper but devoid of heart and soul. Each time my students read aloud their seven page psychotherapy code of ethics, I watch them go into their heads, space out, be overwhelmed, and get generally discouraged.

Notice whether or not you have any of the following responses when you read or hear the words: "Code of Ethics."

confusion	guilt or shame
self-righteousness	dismissal of value
freezing or dissociating	excessively detailed questioning
paranoia or fear	tightening up
overwhelm	boredom
discouragement or frustration	annoyance

Approaching a code of ethics with any of these above responses will obviously interfere with your ability to use the code's potent wisdom and guidance as a resource. First you will need to disengage interfering responses and engage new responses such as relaxing and feeling curious and centered. Being cognitively and emotionally engaged is a first step towards a shift away from habitual responses.

There are situations that are described in ethical codes that may not be in your present awareness as potentially harmful or dynamically and ethically complex. Studying your ethical code, will offer an opportunity to use precision and objectivity in a calm way. This enables you to be more informed thus having more choices for how to respond.

Other challenges

Ways people behave when faced with regulations and rules:

- naive (i.e., just thinking you're a good person is not enough)
- obsessive (i.e., excessive self-watchfulness)
- harmful (i.e., following the letter but not the intention of the law)
- paranoid (fear-based response resulting in being over cautious)
- over-focused on not causing harm to an extent that it interferes with noticing and resolving difficulties
- "How could he have?!" (i.e. disregarding aspiration, intention, mistakes)
- rigid (i.e. dissociating from noticing and caring about personal impact)
- deliberately disobeying (i.e. believing that rules are from a less-evolved system)

Seven Principles

A commonly-referenced set of seven principles comes from Redlich and Pope (1980). These principles are helpful in providing a simple overview of the territory of ethics. With this preface, a many-page detailed code can be less daunting. *"These are (1) above all, do no harm; (2) practice only with competence; (3) do not exploit; (4) treat people with respect for their dignity as human beings; (5) protect confidentiality; (6) act, except in the most extreme instances, only after obtaining informed consent; and (7) practice, insofar as possible, within the framework of social equity and justice."* [xx]

Summary of Categories

Here is a summary of categories and behavioral expectations common to most codes. This is a condensed and simplified list that covers most everyday situations helping professionals encounter. This chapter is not a replacement for detailed study of your particular ethical code.

Level of Competence

- practice only in ways and areas in which the practitioner is competent
- maintain competency and stay current with new developments
- make appropriate referrals when needed
- handle termination in such a way that client does not feel abandoned
- make an accurate and truthful representation of credentials

Record Keeping

- keep appropriate records of services for legal and consultation purposes
- hold all records in strict confidence

Professional Responsibility

- know, understand, and abide by the code of ethics and legislation on all levels regarding the profession
- conform to generally accepted standards of practice
- use non-exploitative business practices
- avoid discredit to the profession
- properly report potential or actual dangers with both clients and colleagues

Sexuality

- do not become sexually involved with a client

Boundaries

- be responsible for maintaining all appropriate boundaries

Confidentiality

- safeguard all information obtained while providing service, including the fact that the client is a client

- obtain the informed written consent of client (with some exceptions)
- adequately disguise any confidential information used for teaching or research so as to prevent client identification
- hold information in confidence even after the professional relationship ends
- use appropriate legal or professional disclosure statements

Ethical Codes also contain information about potential dilemmas that require complex understanding of relationship dynamics, laws and legal ramifications, and considerations of the impact on clients over time. Detailed guidance about these complex situations is readily available through written documentation.

Issues Getting Further Study and Refinement

The following are several contemporary ethical issues that are currently under consideration and further study by some professional organizations. The American Psychological Association (APA), for example, describes the APA Ethics Code as "based on day-to-day decisions made by psychologists in the practice of their profession, rather than prescribed by a committee."[xxi] It is important to keep up to date with these as they receive more attention and refinement. Take time to check your profession's guidelines for these issues, and apply your felt sense of the effect of the power differential in these areas:

- dual role relationships
- therapeutic use of touch
- how to respond to possible unethical behavior by a colleague[xxii]
- diversity and multi-cultural issues
- use of technology, internet, email and social media

Technology

Ethical issues related to technology cover therapy using distance technologies such as telephone, SKYPE and Facetime, and audio and video recording; use of electronic communication like email; and use of social media for marketing and for connecting.

Aspects of concern focus on confidentiality and informed consent, multiple relationships, boundaries between our professional and personal lives, and appropriate use in therapy.

In the use of email with clients, talking about risks and expectations is a crucial foundation. Drude and Lichstein offer a detailed discussion of multiple considerations.[xxiii]

Distance therapy possibilities invite ethical thinking about what kinds of clients or client issues are or are not appropriate, and what kinds of email communications are useful between therapist and client. Electronic communication is notably easily misinterpreted.

These questions [about social media] are really interesting because they are pushing us to think clearly about the relationship between our professional and personal lives. We all have our own social communities and networks, but we also have to be aware about how we act and what we disclose in those domains that are more accessible. APA's Ethics Director, Stephen Behnke, discusses technology ethics as an evolving field in which we are now assessing potential harm in order to offer protective guidance.[xxiv]

Misuse of power against oneself

There is another issue that should be in ethical codes and guidelines--practitioners should be aware of and refrain from misusing their power against themselves. We misuse power against ourselves when we are overly critical, when we don't take care of ourselves, when we push ourselves too hard (or not enough), when we can't forgive ourselves, and when we can't let go.

Challenging Issues

Ethical codes are a continually evolving set of guidelines for beneficent professional behavior. One way of looking at this evolution is research. A study by Pope, Tabachnick, and Keith-Spiegel used a questionnaire filled out by "*a national sample of psychologists regarding the degree to which they engaged in each of 83 behaviors and the degree to which they considered each behavior to be ethical. Examples of the 83 behaviors are: treating homosexuality per se as pathological; accepting a client's decision to commit suicide; discussing clients (without names) with friends; engaging in sexual fantasies about a client; going into business with a client; breaking confidentiality if a client is suicidal; charging a client no fee; making a custody evaluation without seeing both parents; hugging a client; signing for hours a supervisee has not earned; filing an ethics complaint against a colleague; performing forensic work for a contingency fee; altering a diagnosis to meet insurance criteria; breaking confidentiality to report child abuse; inviting clients to a party or social event; accepting goods as payment; seeing a minor client without parental consent; telling a client "I'm sexually attracted to you"; terminating therapy if a client cannot pay; asking favors from clients; using a law suit to collect fees; lending money to a client; becoming sexually involved with a former client; and engaging in sex with clinical supervisees.*[xxv]   The behaviors in this list are behaviors that many therapists engage in and no longer consider not to be unethical or are unsure about their ethicality. Is it okay to give a client a hug? Is it ever okay to accept a gift? When is it okay to self-disclose?   Can sexual attraction be talked about as a therapeutic issue? Can some dual role relationships be therapeutically helpful? These are examples of issues that will be re-examined in terms of their probability of causing harm.

There is more information about these issues in following chapters of this book. The internet is becoming a more and more useful, up-to-date, diverse, and efficient resource for staying current and going into more depth about issues of interest. As they say, "just google it."

Remember that circumstances happen in which, even with our best intentions; and even when we know and understand the code of ethics, we make mistakes. Our impact doesn't match our intention, we misunderstand or are misunderstood, or we were unaware of the potential for harm. The best strategy for preventing the escalation of harm is to be proactive about tracking for and resolving relationship difficulties as close to their occurrence as possible.

> *Ethics may, in truth, be the inner, wiser self that guides us in ever more civilized society as we grow beyond our more primitive responses coming from fear and the heady challenges of grandiosity. In a state of confident fearlessness, I suspect that we are far better able to use power for the benefit of others. Ethical codes and guidelines give us a standard to reach for. Having a conceptual framework, allows us to measure our power responses against them and to gain in our skill in applying power in life situations. In very demanding situations, we usually rely on our first impulses, so those impulses should be informed by our knowledge of the coded wisdom of the profession. —Anna Cox.*[xxvi]

> *"Ethics are an essential guide for the work of therapy [and other service professions]. They are a process through which we awaken, enhance, inform, expand, and improve our ability to respond effectively to those who come to us for help."*
> *—Pope and Vasquez*[xxvii]

Self-Study: What's Your Felt Sense?

1. Rewiring
Take a few minutes to identify any habitual personal responses to written codes of ethics that interfere with your ability to use your code as the resource that it is meant to be. Now imagine rewiring your internal connections so that you can now respond in a calm, relaxed, interested, and resourced way.

2. What's Your Felt Sense?
Since the impact of the power differential is the foundation for most codes and guidelines, try out using what you have just learned to understand what the possible client harm is in each of these situations:

- Engaging in a dual role relationship.
- Responding to a client who expresses concern about you and asks you how you are.
- Working with a client from another culture.
- Working with trauma when you have no specific training.
- Responding to a client who gives you a gift.
- Responding to a client's request to be a Facebook friend.

3. What's New?
As you re-read your Code of Ethics, notice if there is anything you don't understand or that is new or surprising information. Clarify what you don't understand with a supervisor or colleague. Discuss what is new or surprising.

4. Misusing Power Against Yourself
Identify and describe a time when you misused your power against yourself and the impact that it had on you. Is this habitual or a one-time event? What kind of repair can you make? How can you interrupt this habit in the future?

5. Remember
Remember with satisfaction a time when you used your power skillfully and either prevented or repaired harm with one of your clients.

Confidentiality

Professional confidentiality is the commitment to keep personal information about clients private. Confidentiality is the foundation for safety, privacy, and self-revelation for clients of psychotherapists and other helping professionals. The confidentiality agreement conveys respect, elicits trust, and offers protection for your client's spirit. Without it, clients may be unable to do the vulnerable work of healing and transformation that they have come to you for.

It is a caregiver's duty to keep personal information confidential except in certain circumstances as required by law, or with the permission of the client.

Duty to Report

Duty to Report (or Duty to Warn and Protect) is the civic requirement that therapists report to appropriate authorities, client situations in which they have assessed

- abuse and/or neglect to a child under 18
- imminent, life-threatening danger to or by the client to self or another identifiable person
- (in many states) abuse and/or neglect of disabled or dependent adults or elders

Confidentiality is protected by law, but when there is imminent danger, confidentiality agreements are overridden. Duty to Report issues usually arise suddenly, so it is important to have thought through your options ahead of time so you can take ethical action in the moment.

Clients should be told about the limits of confidentiality before they disclose private information. It is not ethical or fair to explain mandatory reporting to a client after they have revealed a reportable incident. They should understand and agree to the limitations of confidentiality without coercion before beginning therapy.

Informed Consent

An informed consent form should be signed at the beginning of therapy and should include verbal, or preferably written information about:

- your training and how you work
- supervision
- confidentiality limits (see below)
- discussion and guidelines about touch (if used)
- your fees and collection policies
- how you keep records
- cancellation policies
- phone calls between sessions
- termination process

Additional Disclosures

Additional Disclosures you may wish to make specifically referring to confidentiality include: (Check your state statutes for specifics. This one is aligned with the statutes in Colorado.)

The information you discuss during a psychotherapy session is protected as confidential under law with certain limitations.

It is my policy to report suspected child abuse to the proper authorities who may then investigate.

I also may take some action without your consent if I deem you to be a serious harm to yourself or another. Any action I take without your consent will be discussed with you.

If I am unable to collect my agreed upon fee, I may send your name and address to a collection agency.

If you file an official complaint or a lawsuit against me, your right to confidentiality will be waived.

If you choose to use your health benefit plan, with your consent your insurance company or managed care company will require confidential information to determine eligibility for reimbursement.

I may seek consultation from another mental health professional. However, your identity will not be revealed without your consent, and your privacy will be protected by that professional.

I hire a person to do my billing, and she has access to limited confidential information, for example, your name and address, diagnosis, and dates of sessions. This information is protected from further disclosure and is used solely for billing purposes.

In the event that you choose to use your health care benefits and my services are reimbursable under your insurance plan, you will have to give me consent to release required information. Released confidential information may range from identifying information, diagnosis, and dates of sessions to a complete assessment with treatment goals and progress reports when your benefits fall under managed care. In some instances, I may have a contract with the third party payer that requires me to submit confidential information and to have my psychotherapy with you managed by the agent company of the insurance company. I can not be in control of the storage of confidential information nor access to your confidential information when it is given to a third party. The insurance company will determine benefit coverage and the kind of service for which they will reimburse. I will discuss with you my recommendations for treatment, and you will decide how you want to proceed.

Release of Information

A release of information form should state as specifically as possible what information is to be released and to whom. The disclosure should be limited to only those persons and to only that content considered necessary by professional standards for dealing with the particular situation. "Blanket" or non-specific releases are not ethical and may not provide sufficient legal protection. In section 1.07C of the NASW Code of Ethics[xxviii] (and this is common to other codes), Social Workers are required to "disclose the least amount of confidential information necessary to achieve the desired purpose." Psychotherapists need to insure that they have their clients' permission to release information, and a signed release is a documentation of that fact. Verbal permission is okay in many situations but should be noted in your client records. Confidential information used for teaching or research needs to be adequately disguised to prevent client identification.

This is a sample release form.

Release of Confidential Information
Therapist's name
Address
Phone/Email

    I,_____
authorize _____ to disclose
to _____ the following information:
_____
for the following purpose(s): _____.

    I understand that my records are protected under federal and state regulations and cannot be disclosed without my express written consent unless otherwise provided for in the regulations. I also understand that I may revoke this consent at any time, and that in any event this consent expires automatically as described below. I understand that the person or agency requesting this information may not transfer any information it may receive without obtaining written permission to do so.

    Date, event or condition upon which this consent expires:
_____
Client signature _____ date _____
Therapist signature _____ date _____

Within the framework that protective privilege ends where the public peril begins, therapists and helping professionals often have choices about HOW to most effectively and supportively honor the protective duty to report.

In your power differential role, you must use your best judgment about how to protect your client's spirit and prevent or reduce harm. You may need to make judgment calls about:

- the seriousness and imminence of the possible harm
- the intent and impact of an ethical violation (i.e. willful and repetitive, or naïve and unintended)
- whether the alleged violation occurred or was a projection.

These are often "tough calls" to make and supervision is of great help.

Situations to Consider

1. Your new client tells you that her former partner is now dating their former therapist. This former therapist is a colleague whom you know personally.

Whenever you have information about possible ethical violations by a colleague, you have a professional responsibility to take action through appropriate channels. If your information comes from a client, you need written permission from your client to talk with your colleague unless you feel "disclosure is necessary to prevent serious, foreseeable, and imminent harm" (Social Workers Code of Ethics 1.07.C[xxix])

You could file a grievance with a grievance board and let them investigate this, but it is generally recommended that you first speak directly and constructively with your colleague about your concerns. The information you get from this conversation would then assist you in assessing how to proceed depending on your assessment related to truth, imminence, and intent, as described above. Supervision could be very helpful at this point.

2. A colleague comes to you for a peer consultation and tells you that he/she is having a sexual liaison with a client.

Assessment question: How willing is this colleague to take responsibility, self-correct, and repair the situation?

3. Your teenage client comes in with visible bruises, saying that his father hit him again. Your client is afraid that if you report this to social services, he will be put into foster care.

Assessment question: How can you attend to your clients fear about losing his father and protect your client from further abuse?

4. Your client reports that several years ago, he abused his child. Your client feels that he has now worked through this and it hasn't happened again, but he needs to unburden himself and work with his shame about it.

Assessment question: How well do you know your client and can you be sure that the abuse is not current?

5. Your client talks about being angry with her spouse. Your client describes fantasies of being violent.

Assessment question: How well do you know your client? Is she working on learning to express anger appropriately, or does she have a history of uncontrolled anger.

6. Your client is contemplating suicide.

Assessment question: How specific and imminent is the contemplation?

7. You are working with a couple, and the husband reveals in a private session, that he is currently having an affair and is not intending to tell his wife but knows he can tell you this because of your confidentiality agreement.

Assessment question: How could you clarify the difference here between confidentiality and unhealthy and harmful secrecy?

8. A 19-year-old woman is referred to you for counseling by her mother who is very concerned about her well-being. After several sessions with the daughter, the mother calls you to see how things are going and insists on your opinion since she is paying for the sessions.

Assessment questions: What kind of consent do you need? How can you respond to the concerns of the Mom in a supportive way?

General Principles

Here are some general principles for making assessments and judgment calls in situations such as described above:

- Trust your ability to perceive accurately and use your knowledge of your client or colleague's past behaviors.
- Ask your clients direct questions about the seriousness and imminence of their intentions. Tell them what you are thinking or feeling and the choices available. Make it clear that you want to act with their safety and best interests in mind.
- Make every effort to support your client or colleague in reporting to the appropriate authorities about the situation. Stay in the room while the call is made.
- Attempt to find a course of action that will not only prevent or reduce harm but promote your client's well-being and personal empowerment.
- Take charge and take strong action when the situation is urgent. This may actually help your client feel safer and model setting limits.
- Don't make confidentiality agreements that support unhealthy or harmful secrets.
- Keep a list in your office of contact information for authorities and resources.

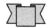

- Keep appropriate written agreements and records, and document your actions in situations that are challenging or easily misconstrued.

Confidentiality is one of the most complex and challenging issues facing therapists and helping professionals. In working with confidentiality dilemmas, you have an opportunity to sensitively use your power to either keep or disclose private information, while meeting the legal requirements, and continuing to support the therapeutic relationship. In doing this your client's self-esteem and empowerment also gets supported.

Self-Study: Options

1. Think through the situations described in the "situations to consider" section to identify several possible courses of action for your choice of three of these.

Dual Role Relationships

Story: *A therapist had been a long-time member of a dynamic singing group. One of his clients showed up at a rehearsal very eager to join. In their next therapy session, the client expressed great excitement about singing together. The therapist talked about his concern that the power differential would affect their therapeutic relationship. He asked his client to think about how it would be to be in the singing group and then to meet each week in this confidential, therapeutic relationship that focused on her. How, he wondered aloud, would it be for her to see him in both these contexts? After some thought, she said, "Oh my, I am so relieved that you understand about these dynamics! I thought I was being WEIRD to feel uncomfortable about it. I appreciate talking about it directly. I think I'll find another group to sing with. I'm sorry because I love your group, but I just think it wouldn't work."*

A dual role relationship is any additional relationship with a client or student occurring simultaneously with the therapy or educational relationship, or with a previous therapy or educational relationship. The impact of the power differential is what makes these relationships problematic and challenging.

Ordinary, everyday boundary crossings such as a chance meeting in the grocery store, attendance at a church service, being at the same party, seeing a client at a concert are not considered dual role relationships because they do not involve new roles and they are not on-going relationships. These meetings can be simply managed by a practical protocol of acknowledging each other and leaving it to your client to name your professional relationship if he or she chooses.

Multiple role relationships are prohibited or discouraged in ethical codes. However, in small and/or interwoven communities, some dual roles are often unavoidable. The 1993 American Psychological Association Code of Ethics[xxx] recognizes that when consciously managed and not exploitative, they are not necessarily harmful (with the exception of sexual relationships and offering a commission or reward to clients for referring other clients to you.)

A different term—"Undue Influence" replaces the category Dual Role Relationship in the Colorado Association of Psychotherapists Code of Ethics[xxxi]. Recognizing that dual role relationships occur in any size community, this terminology appropriately focuses attention toward the potential client harm from undue influence rather than on prohibiting multiple role relationships. This code says simply: *"Members shall not enter into a therapeutic relationship with a client where there is undue influence to the detriment of the client. Members shall be especially sensitive to conflicts of interest that may arise from dual relationships during or immediately before or after a therapeutic relationship."* When a dual role relationship is determined to have low risk of undue influence, there are guidelines (some listed here) for consciously, honestly, openly, and attentively managing this relationship.

Generally, the effect of dual role relationships is some level of dependency on the therapist for emotional warmth, support, and inclusion, and this dependency is set within, created, and maintained by the power differential inherent in the therapist/client roles.

> *My colleague, Anna Cox*[xxxii] *adds, "Because of the power differential in therapy settings, the therapist may often not realize the amount of energy that is invested in them and in their role. Although inescapable in the therapy setting and sometimes helpful as a therapeutic tool, this power differential makes a client very vulnerable to the therapist outside the safety of the therapy office. A casual word or action by the therapist that would not likely cause notice by those not in therapy with them, could cause great pain to a client...The therapist can be harmed as well because there are many levels of misperception possible. In states of distress the client could hurt the therapist professionally by damaging their reputation or by making accusations.*

The most frequent exception to this is when the client is also a colleague in the healing field, or when the non-therapeutic relationship has a low level of intimacy (although this level of equality also needs to be managed).

Types of Dual Role Relationships
The following would be considered multiple role relationships:
* friendship
* business or financial

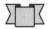

- barter
- serving together on a committee
- being an administrator or supervisor to your client
- being a colleague, supervisor, or student of your client in another arena
- being in a staff group or professional peer group
- sexual (current or previous)
- rewarding clients to solicit other clients
- consistent activities in political, social, or religious groups
- loaning money
- attending workshops and trainings

Relationships between graduate students or assistants and educators

Ofer Zur,[xxxiii] renowned ethics expert in psychology, offers insight into the special category of training relationships. As he puts it, *"unlike client-therapist relationships, training relationships are intrinsically multifaceted and by their nature consist of overlapping roles with various expectations, responsibilities, and obligations. For instance, faculty members are not only responsible for imparting knowledge and evaluating students on that knowledge, but typically also serve as advisors, supervisors, and mentors for students. Faculty members tend to play a role in hiring students for assistantships and in selecting students for awards, scholarships, grants, and professional opportunities. Additionally, it is not uncommon for faculty members and students to work together on research projects, co-author articles/presentations, and interact in professional and social settings outside of the immediate training environment. Each of these roles entails various obligations and responsibilities that have the potential to be in competition with one another."* These situations can create stress and confusion for students or training assistants. Awareness, sensitivity and good communication in managing these multiple roles will go a long way in reducing anxiety and increasing clarity.

Dual Role Factors and Considerations
Dual role relationships can be the source of serious ethical and relationship problems. In the State of Colorado, grievances about dual relationships are in the top third of those filed. You will need to be impeccably clear about boundaries and on-going communication, in managing a multiple role relationship.

Here are some factors to consider in deciding if a possible dual relationship could become problematic.

*   whether the practitioner has any kind of evaluative function, i.e. grading, assessing performance, hiring or firing
*   length of time between the therapeutic relationship and any other relationship, if the dual role would not be concurrent
*   whether the exchange of goods and/or services would be contra-indicated or exploitive
*   the nature and frequency of the dual function or role
*   the degree of intimacy involved in the professional relationship (generally the greater the intimacy, the greater the need for caution)
*   the nature and seriousness of the client's problem and kind of therapy used
*   the stage in therapy process: beginning, middle, or end (generally, the earlier the stage, the greater the need for caution)
*   the ability to keep the two relationships separate—client's ability, practitioner's ability, and the capacity for the practitioner/client system to handle the two relationships.
*   level of maturity and communication skills of both parties

A Legal Statute

Here is a representative legal statute for showing evidence when engaging in a dual role. The Colorado Mental Health Statutes Rule 10,[xxxiv] states:

> *"Any supervisor or psychotherapist claiming an exception to the code violation prohibiting dual relationships due to practice in a rural location, cultural community, accredited training institution of formal learning, or special needs to the clinical population being served. . . .shall show by a preponderance of the evidence:*
>
> *The client was fully informed of the dual relationship and the possibilities for conflicts of interest;*
>
> *The client's access to quality care has not been compromised;*
>
> *The supervisor and psychotherapist have not benefited from the relationship over and above a reasonable fee for service (i.e., that the power in the therapeutic relationship has not been used to influence the therapeutic relationship for personal gain);*

The therapeutic and supervisory relationships have not been compromised and the best interests of the client are served by the relationship."

Reasons to Discourage[xxxv]

Here are some reasons to discourage dual role relationships:
* It is considered undue influence when the practitioner has any kind of evaluative function. Thus dual role relationships where there is an evaluative function are generally unmanageable.
* The client can be more easily and deeply hurt by an unintended gesture or comment.
* The client may be consciously or unconsciously afraid of being judged or evaluated.
* The counselor may not be as confrontive with the clients they see in other roles. The therapist's own need to be liked and accepted may lead them to be less challenging.
* Dual relationships tend to impair the therapist's judgment.
* The possibility of exploiting the client is more likely when the relationship takes on social dimensions.
* There is potential for conflict of interest.
* The client may become inhibited in therapy due to fear of losing the relationship. The client may fear losing respect, or being excluded by the therapist, and thus may censor disclosures, and find it difficult to be honest about their feelings (especially negatives ones) in the relationship.
* Blurred boundaries can distort the professional nature of the therapeutic relationship.
* The therapist may have the adulation of the client. When there is a dual relationship, a "fall from grace" may be especially confusing, difficult, and personal, instead of primarily role-related.
* Client may have unconscious expectations that the (former) therapeutic contract takes precedence over the new relationship.

Barter Considerations

Here are some additional considerations about bartering:
* Bartering is discouraged in most codes of ethics and prohibited in some. In some cases, this may be the only way for a client to get the help they need. Some therapists provide their service free or at a reduced rate, and instead of bartering, ask that the client engage in volunteer service for a community organization as a trade.

- Barter has great potential for conflict.
- The client can become resentful when expected to provide several hours of work for one hour of therapy.
- The therapist may resent the client if the work for trade (such as car repair, gardening, house cleaning) is not done properly, and the client can then suffer from this resentment. The therapist can be critical of the client's work.
- Clients can be put in a bind if they learn certain personal information about their therapist.
- The therapist may manipulate or influence the client to provide better services.

Here are some situations in which multiple role relationships caused harm to clients. These are actual grievances.[xxxvi]

"A clinician develops a relationship with a client, both in individual and group therapy. During this period, the client and therapist also begin a social relationship, meeting for coffee, walks, and a holiday party at the therapist's home. The therapist also hires the client to assist in the development of a healing arts related business. The same clinician allows a different client to live at the therapist's residence while the client/therapist relationship is ongoing.

"A therapist begins working as a "business coach' for a particular company, helping employees become organized. AT the same time, the clinician begins providing marriage and family therapy to company employees. Several company employees who are both being 'coached' and in treatment with the clinician believe themselves to be in a confidential relationship and make personal and confidential disclosures to the therapist. The information learned by the therapist is subsequently relayed to third parties, including family members and co-workers, unbeknownst to the client/employee."

Safeguards
These are some safeguard choices that could be used when entering into and managing a dual role relationship.
- Contemplate and sense what the additional relationship might be like. Try it on in your mind and see how it feels.
- Secure the client's informed consent.
- Discuss the potential risks and benefits of dual relationship.
- Continue to assess and discuss the impact throughout the course of the relationship.

- Consult with other professionals to resolve dilemmas.
- Get supervision when the risk for harm is high.
- Document the dual relationship in case notes.
- Carefully examine and re-examine motives of both parties.
- Create a personal process for roling and de-roling.
- Delineate boundaries on time, space, payment, and purpose very clearly.
- Be available and non-defensive if or when the client brings up a problem. Take the initiative to talk about concerns that arise.
- Remember that, although you are both equally responsible (100%), you, as the one with the greater role power, are more responsible (150%).

Managing Dual Role Relationships

Sometimes I employ organizers for my programs who have been students of mine in the past. As part of our contracting for our new roles, I ask, "How will it be for you to have this new role with me?" One woman said, "I'm sure it will be just fine, but frankly, I can't even imagine what I should watch out for. Can you tell me what problems could come up?" Based on this conversation, I made the following list that is now a document in include in my negotiations. Perhaps it will be useful to you.

The items on this list are things that are specifically for the person shifting out of a down-power role. The list is particularly useful because these responses are difficult if not impossible to predict in advance. Keep in mind that the person in the up-power role in the prior relationship bears 150% responsibility for tracking and attending to the new relationship. Also note that these items are things for both parties to watch out for and bring up. As with most relationship maintenance, the sooner a concern is brought up, the more creatively and effectively it can be attended to. Regular check-ins even when there is no concern is of preventive value.

Things to watch out for and name when choosing to be in a multiple role relationship:

- resentment or feeling taken advantage of
- wanting or attempting to take care of the other at your own expense
- feeling disempowered
- trying to do it all too perfectly
- feeling abnormally guilty, wrong, or at fault
- feeling surprised or confused by some behavior of the other
- feeling unclear about responsibilities that accompany each role
- feeling confused about when and how to be in each role, and how to shift from one to another
- feeling uncertain or burdened by a new level of sharing personal information
- feeling strongly vulnerable or young or incompetent
- being unsure or unclear about mutual agreements or contracts
- discovering assumed expectations based on the other or previous role relationship

An outdoor wilderness program staff uses a contract as part of their management of the following dual role relationship. This is an excerpt from a larger document.*xxxvii* *"As support staff, for a program in which my primary partner chooses to enroll, I am aware of the inherent "power differential" that is created. I have discussed this power differential with the Guides for this program and with my partner. I understand the following measures and agreements have been formulated to best support the safety of all participants and staff; to minimize the impact of the power differential; and to honor and protect me, my partner and the integrity of the program. Agreements: 1. I agree to meet with the Guides and my partner prior to program to discuss how the container will be held. 2. I agree to acknowledge to all participants the presence of my dual relationship with one of the participants from the very beginning of the program. 3. I agree to pay close attention to the very "subtle" ways that the following issues may show up and bring these issues to the awareness of the Guides should they arise. a) I agree to not show favoritism toward my partner over other participants through my words, actions or attention. b) I agree to hold in confidence all information concerning my partner and other participants that is discussed during staffing. d) I agree to track my interactions with my partner and watch for any ways in which these interactions might interfere with my partner doing her "work". f) I agree to follow up with the Guides a couple of weeks after the program and address any concerns that may have arisen. g) I agree to not have physical intimacy with my partner beginning 24 hours prior to start of program and until program is complete.*

Successful managing of dual role relationships that are necessary or deemed to have less risk of undue influence, seem to depend on boundaries, vulnerability and communication.

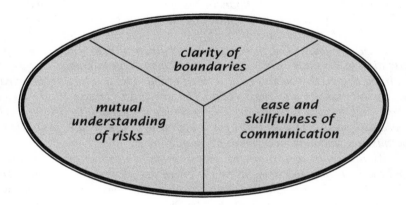

Here's a example of using these three considerations in deciding how to manage the roles.

Story: *A colleague describes this successful management of dual roles: "I am the only body centered experiential therapist in town with many graduate psychology students in my caseload. The Psychology program at the University invited me to teach a graduate course on body centered therapy. I wanted to teach this course, but it would mean being both therapist and teacher for a subgroup of students. As a win/win resolution to this dilemma, I co-taught the course with a professor who gave assignments and graded the papers and exams. This way I did not execute judgment (grading them) on therapy clients for their work as students. Also, I asked each of the grad-student clients about the upcoming dual relationship a priori and ongoingly processed this during the dual relationship period. In retrospect: It went well. Clients made leaps of personal growth via class assignments. Factors for this turning out well were: clarity about boundaries surrounding this event, the time-*

limitedness, and ongoing openness and processing about the effect of the dual role relationship."

Story: *This is a situation in which the dual roles did not work out well and the client unfortunately experienced significant harm. Client and therapist had a long, intense, and successful therapeutic relationship. Both were psychotherapists in the same community. Both wanted to take the same professional year-long training. The therapist registered for a similar training in another town to avoid the dual role. However, some personal issues made it difficult to take that training. So, she asked her client how she would feel about her taking the local training, citing her own chronic health and financial issues. Because of the increased influence of the power differential and the client's history of sacrificing her own needs to take care of family members, the client said "yes" to the therapist's request. The therapist wanted to hear "yes" and didn't pay attention to the client's history and ambivalent body language. Before the training began, they made, what seemed at the time, a reasonable contract to try to manage the dual roles. The therapist agreed to do a free additional therapy session after each monthly weekend of the training. The therapist had acknowledged the dual roles, asked for her client's permission, and made a contract for managing it.*

As the Training progressed, however, both the therapy relationship and the learning environment for the client got progressively worse. This client had felt manipulated into acquiescing even though she was uncomfortable and concerned, by the expressed personal needs of the therapist. She had repeated an old pattern of taking care of an authority figure in order not to lose love. Working with this pattern had been her main therapy goal. She felt compromised in her participation in the training, becoming less and less of herself as more and more of her energy went into handling feeling "triggered," managing her feelings toward the therapist and avoiding classroom situations that would put her in direct contact with the therapist. The therapist did not initiate checking in about how the dual relationship was going, and the pre-training agreement did not address what would happen if it was not working out. Difficult situations that emerged during the training for this client included such things as handling seeing her therapist working as a client, overlapping friendships, social occasions, and competition for future teaching opportunities. This therapist was unable to understand the many ways in which she had misused her power, although she did admit that "she had become simple-minded and only able to think of this person as a colleague and not as her client." The situation was not successfully resolved.

Looking at dilemmas by focusing on **both** preventing harm and promoting learning, provides opportunities for creative solutions in working effectively with dual roles that can't be avoided or that can be well-managed through good boundaries and communication.

Self-study practice: What Could Be Managed?

Now, given all these guidelines and statutes, how would this actually work? Here is a collection of possible situations. Take a look at them and, using the information above, write in the situation numbers that you would guess to be most likely to have that outcome. For each situation, identify the factors that would influence your decision.

work out well _____
be a disaster _____
be challenging to manage _____
be relatively easy to manage _____
don't go there _____

1. You are a teacher and your students invite you to have lunch with them.
What factors would enter into your decision?

2. Your client is a student in a Masters program in psychotherapy. He/she must do 30 sessions of personal therapy and mentoring to get degree. At end of 30 sessions, client initiates a friendship.
What factors would enter into your decision?

3. You have enrolled as a marketer for some vitamins that you are very impressed by and have heard stories of miraculous healings. You think these vitamins would be just the right thing for this particular client.
What factors would enter into your decision?

4. You and your client have a good connection during massage work. Your client, after the 5th session, invites you to their birthday party saying that it is very important to them to have their closest friends there. You personally are new to the area and are trying to enlarge your social circle.
What factors would enter into your decision?

5. You have been doing very good work with a client and things are progressing well. Your client loses her job and can no longer pay you. They offer to trade for doing bookkeeping for you.

What factors would enter into your decision?

6. Your client seems to be feeling attracted to you and wants to get together for lunch.

What factors would enter into your decision?

7. You need more clients and think about offering a free session to any client who refers someone to you.

What factors would enter into your decision?

8. One of your clients wants to enroll in a weekend course that you are teaching.

What factors would enter into your decision?

9. You discover that one of your clients has just joined a choir that you have been singing with for years.

What factors would enter into your decision?

10. One of the therapists you supervise is teaching a class you would like to take.

What factors would enter into your decision?

11. Your client offers to pay ahead for sessions so that you can cover some unpaid debt.

What factors would enter into your decision?

12. A previous lover calls to do therapy with you.

What factors would enter into your decision?

13. You meet your client at a party. *How do you handle this?*

14. You live in a small community in which you do massage with the same person who is your job supervisor in the kitchen.

How do you handle this?

15. You are a volunteer working for an environmental organization and a client gets elected to the Board of Directors.

What factors would enter into your decision?

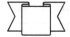

Ethical Decision-Making

The basic ethical question: **Is what I am doing in the best interest of my client?** (Or my student, or supervisee, or colleague, or employee?) With this question in mind, there are two kinds of ethical decision-making requiring ethical attention—ordinary moment ethical decision-making and more complex ethical decision-making. Both kinds are essential to deepening trust and being in right relationship. Both involve an integration of personal integrity with professional responsibility. Commitment to the best interests of your clients is the often unnamed and yet constant foundation that guides your interventions.

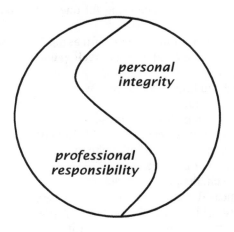

Ordinary Moment Ethical Decision-making

I find that we as professionals most often think of ethical decision-making simply and solely as the complex type described below without putting conscious attention toward our ordinary, everyday kind of ethical decision-making. However, the great preponderance of ethical decisions are actually made moment to moment in the ordinary process of being of service to your clients. These require integrity, compassion, tracking subtle energetic cues and attunement to being in right relationship. Here are some everyday, normal ethical decision-making instances using ordinary client questions:

How often should I be coming to see you?

Will you write a recommendation for me?

Can we go later today?

Can I pay at a reduced rate?

Would you meet me for coffee to talk about a business idea?

Is this situation I'm in a healthy one?

Would you tell me about your marriage?

I brought you a gift.

Could you visit me at my home?

What should I do? Please tell me. I can't figure it out myself.

Responding to questions like these happens in the moment. You don't have time to ask your supervisor or to consult your ethical code. Many of these issues aren't even covered by a specific rule or guideline. To respond you have to go to your gut feeling, your humanity, your curiosity, and to your felt sense of the relationship. The right or ethical answer to each of these questions could be one thing for one client and the opposite for another client.

Other ordinary moment ethical decision-making happens moment-to-moment based on your trained and personal feeling about

what's needed next,

how much to lead and how much to follow,

what particular technique to use,

when to do nothing but be lovingly present,

when to share in your experience of the dilemma of being human,

when to include your client in what you're thinking,

when to offer advice or guidance,

how to respond to challenging feedback or anger.

This is truly ethical decision-making as right use of your power and influence in the relationship in which you have up-power authority. Once again, ethics is relational. Ethics is about caring about the impact you have on others.

In our rushed and speeded up lives and work environments, it's easy to get caught or distracted by the need for instant responses, instant action, efficiency, compartmentalizing, and multi-tasking. Ethics in the ordinary moments, however, requires slowing down and being present, caring, and thoughtful. *"It is when we slow down that we show up."*[xxxviii] This is ethics from the inside out, rather than the rule side in. The majority of this book

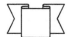

focuses on helping you fine-tune your sensitivity and awareness toward ethical decision-making of the ordinary moment kind.

Complex Ethical Decision-making Using Ethical Codes & Power Spiral

Far less frequently, you are called to make complex ethical decisions that require time to think through your response, consulting with your supervisor, referring to your Ethical Code, and/or using the Power Spiral model in this chapter. Even though these moments are less frequent, they certainly not less important! Examples of such ethical challenges might be:

- deciding how to manage an inevitable dual role relationship
- making a DSM5 diagnosis and considering the ramifications
- reporting impending or actual harm effectively and skillfully
- confidentiality exceptions
- deciding whether your client is being re-traumatized
- making appropriate referrals
- responding and adapting to cultural diversity
- use of touch
- self-disclosure
- handling sexual issues
- dealing with possible unethical behavior by colleagues
- whether you are working outside your area of competence
- concerns about suicide, violence or danger to others

There are many excellent ethics courses that cover specific ethical codes in great detail, risk management concerns, and case studies of difficult situations. This book focuses more on ordinary every-day decision-making.

John May[xxxix] describes the need for both rules and sensitivity to each therapeutic relationship:

"Successfully navigating ethical conflicts is not simply a matter of thinking about what you believe is right and then doing it....One needs to know the rules and be able to use them. Some of these rules are more like suggestions or goals to strive for. Others are more like laws, and you need to know them in detail. An analogy would be traffic laws. The difference between a speed limit of 30mph vs. 40mph may not seem like much, but it's enough to get you in trouble. On the other hand, most authors emphasize

that if you go no further than obeying the rules, you are still likely to end up in trouble. . . .Continuing with the analogy to driving, knowing the speed limit, though important, is not enough to make you a good driver. And you are always called to be a good driver. A counselor is likely to encounter a myriad of situations that are not adequately covered by the various ethical codes. The counselor is even likely to encounter occasional situations in which behavior mandated by an ethical code will harm the client. In these situations, the counselor will have to use judgment, brains, maturity, and a deep understanding of ethical behavior to find her way to an ethical resolution of the dilemma."

In these non-ordinary complex situations, there are many forces and influences to consider. Some of these include: regional laws, ethical code, clinical assessment, gut intuition, standards of practice, transference, supervisor recommendations, cultural norms, risk to client and/or caregiver, employer policies, client wishes, client's life circumstances, and your personal issues and feelings.

Some guidelines and considerations

- Involve your client as much as possible in the decision-making. You are making a decision about what is best for your client and including them in the process is empowering and beneficial.
- Keep in mind that your emotions may affect your interpretations and your decision-making.
- Take into consideration your client's values, especially when they differ from your own.
- Document your actions.
- Get support. Your resources may include: the Grievance Board, your supervisor, colleagues, and a lawyer.
- Remember that ethical codes are designed to protect practitioners as well as clients.
- Understand that *"the highest form of caring is the honest expression of benevolence."*[xl]

Professional behavior is devoted to doing no harm. Interestingly, doing no harm can have a subtle and unintended impact of implying that a) it is possible to avoid doing any harm, b) if you inadvertently do cause harm, you should feel ashamed and thus secretive, c) if you apologize or admit fault in any way, this could be used against you and you should and will be punished. These factors may actually discourage taking responsibility for ethical mistakes. More helpful and realistic would be to amend "Do no harm" to: Seek to do no harm and when you cause harm, take responsibility as soon as possible, staying in the relationship and noticing, attending to, and resolving the situation.

Using the Power Spiral

When you have any kind of ethical decision to make, try using the Power Spiral as a resource. You may also find the Power Spiral helpful when you would like to reflect on a decision you made or on a mistake you made (or may have made). Write or think about the situation you want some guidance about. Then place or imagine this situation in the center of the Power Spiral as pictured below. Now imagine sitting in the each of the directions of the Spiral and consider questions such as the ones listed here. What insights do you get?

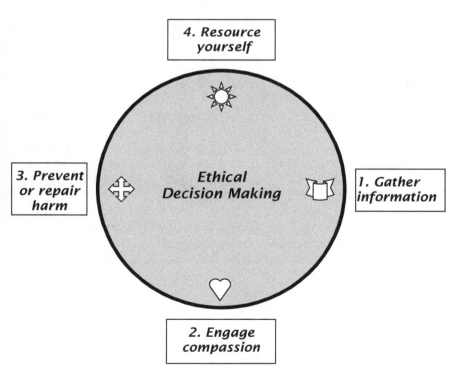

1. Gather information:
— the guided use of power
- What does your code of ethics say about this issue?
- What is the impact of the power differential?
- What other objective information is relevant?

2. Engage compassion:
— the conscious use of power
- How does this issue affect your personally?
- Is shame de-resourcing either you or your client?
- What kind of transference or counter-transference may be operating?

3. Prevent or repair harm:
— the responsible use of power
Some ethical decisions are involved with how to be in service to your client and prevent harm, and others are related to how to resolve difficulties and repair harm.

a) Questions for being of service and preventing harm:
- What are your response options?
- What will be the short and long-term impact of each of these options?
- What additional factors might be important to consider? For example, you could consider other family members, client's life circumstances and abilities, risks to client or therapist, spirit of the law, cultural norms or spiritual beliefs.

b) Questions for resolving difficulties and repairing harm:
- Is there a difference between intention and impact?
- How do you feel toward your client, toward yourself?
- Because of your role, what are you responsible for?
- What is the best strategy for:
  - Compassionately understanding your client's experience and communicating this understanding along with your genuine concern?
  - Ascertaining what kind of repair is needed?
  - Following through in the most appropriate way?

4. Resource yourself:
— the wise use of power

- How will you take care of yourself and use the resources and support available to you?
- How can you use this situation to self-correct and/or be more skillful in the future?
- When you have done all you can, how will you let it go?

Story: *One of my students told me about an experience that usefully illustrates this process. Elena works for an agency. One of her colleagues referred a client to her. The written notes about this client said that he wanted to get disability payments. When she met with David, he said that he didn't want disability assistance. Hearing that and feeling some reticence from David, Elena began working with him on feeling less shame and personal failure at needing to apply for public assistance. This process went nowhere. David stopped coming to appointments and he filed a complaint with Elena's boss. He had quit his appointments because she just wasn't giving him any help with his communication skills and managing his anger. Elena was quite surprised to hear this.*

Using the Power Spiral process, Elena got some insights:

1. That the power differential might have been interfering with David's ability to tell Elena herself the truth that he wasn't getting what he needed. Based on the notes, she had not asked David directly what he wanted help with, assuming his reticence was his discomfort with needing assistance.

2(a). That she was likely projecting her own shame about what it would be like to need public assistance onto David; and (b). that she wasn't checking in with her gut sense of what was going on.

3. That she needed to take responsibility for being insensitive to what David's real needs were and to relying too much on the referral notes she had gotten. She decided her best choice was to make an authentic apology to David and invite him back to work with her on anger and communication skills. Elena also understood that she needed to do some follow-up work with her boss to let him know how the complaint had been successfully handled.

4. Elena took the action she decided on. David did come back to work with Elena on communication and anger and was satisfied with their work. Elena learned to focus on the relationship rather than just the referral notes. She was also happy that she had taken 150% responsibility and reached out to David to resolve and repair.

This is a fairly simple example of how to use the process and the many insights and guidance that the focused questions for each direction can bring. It is also a very humbling example of how easily and innocently we can get off-track. Further, it is a story about how easy it is to be rule-bound (in this case, referral-notes-bound), when we most need to be attuning to ourselves and being in right relationship with our clients--ethics from the inside out. And, finally it is an example of how simple and straightforward it can be to work out a difficulty.

Self-Study Practice: Ordinary and Extraordinary

1. Keeping in mind that ethical decision-making happens in both ordinary, everyday ways and in extraordinary situations: please identify two instances in which, through your attitude, words, or actions, you made an ethical decision—
      a. in an ordinary moment
      b. in a complex situation

2. Think of a personally challenging ethical situation or an ethical decision you have already made that you would like to reflect on. Use the Power Spiral process as described in this chapter to gain additional insight and guidance. You might also consider using this process in a peer supervision group to get further guidance, insight and support from the perspective of colleagues, and to expand the range of considerations and resources you have available to you.

"Always try to do the right thing. It will confound some and gratify the rest."
                                    —*Mark Twain*[xli]

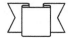

Violations and Statistics

An ethical violation is a behavior defined as a disobeyance of a profession's code of ethics.

A misuse of power is a use of role power that causes client harm or undermines their dignity. This may happen through intimidation, manipulation, shame, exerting undue influence, or disrespect for diversity needs.

Ethical violations and misuses of power are grievable. Grievances may be handled within the relationship or taken to a professional organization, state grievance board, or a court of law. Code violations fit specific categories or may fall into the catch-all category of "services failed to meet generally accepted standards of practice."

Many misuses of power are subtle or unintended but, nevertheless, adversely effect the quality and effectiveness of the professional relationship. **The Right Use of Power approach recommends that the practitioner be alert to the power differential and handle problems within the relationship or through mediation before they escalate into grievances.**

Because of the practitioner's personality or the impact of the power differential, clients may:

• give their consent to misuses of power (*i.e., say yes to touch even when it does not feel appropriate*)

• be naïve, misled, or misinformed about unethical behaviors (*i.e. ask for a dual relationship not knowing the potential dangers*)

• make decisions from a disempowered place (*i.e. agree to more sessions even when they don't feel it is effective*)

When in a position of trust, you are ultimately responsible (150% principle) for the negative impact of your behavior whether this unethical behavior was conscious, unconscious, or a misunderstanding. Maintaining the integrity of the relationship by tracking and attending to inevitable difficulties is an everyday responsibility of helping professionals. The more courageous you are in doing this, the less likely that any problem will escalate. Paying attention and tracking will bring about a more satisfying and effective therapeutic relationship.

I want to also point out that (although you won't be grieved for this) there are numerous ways in which helping professionals misuse power that cause harm to themselves. For example, a habit of always taking all the blame, being overly critical of yourself, or feeling ashamed of small mistakes is a misuse of power against yourself. This can cause you a great deal of unnecessary suffering and leave you disempowered and less effective. Standing in your power makes it easier to be in right relationship with yourself as well as your clients.

***What are the most frequently reported grievances?**[xlii] (listed in order of frequency)*

1. services provided failed to meet generally accepted standards of practice (a catch-all category)*
2. provided services were outside area of competence
3. sexual intimacies with client
4. breach of confidentiality
5. impaired judgment
6. failure to terminate
7. inadequate supervision to supervisees
8. dual relationship with client
9. inadequate or false record keeping
10. failure to refer
11. misrepresented credentials
12. insurance abuse

*Standard of care is a fluid mix of law, licensing regulations, ethical codes, professional consensus, community norms, and the like. It does not require perfection. It is a minimum standard, based on the average practitioner. Careless mistakes or errors of judgment don't put you below the standard of care.[xliii] It is most frequent because it covers a broad range of behaviors. Although this is the most frequent category, it is one that results in many grievance board decisions not to investigate a complaint. Generally, when it is investigated, standard of care is part of a grievance that includes multiple complaints. Examples might be: a therapist who charged for a full session when she didn't see the client for a full session but was covering unbilled phone time; a therapist who made a home visit for a client who was very ill; a therapist who accepted a small gift from her client; or a therapist who was frequently self-disclosing.

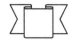

How many therapists actually get grieved and how many lose their licenses?

- In looking at a 1995 study of Colorado therapists by Karla Schmidt,[xliv] I was very curious about how many therapists get grieved and how many lose their licenses. Here's what I discovered: 11% of registered Colorado therapists were grieved in a 6 year period (800 of 7,269), but 77% of these grievances were dismissed.

- Of the 23% of the grievances that were investigated, the Grievance Board "found against" the therapist in 56% of the cases and determined that the therapist was not at fault in 44% of the cases investigated.

- Of the 56% of the cases in which the therapist was "found against," 34% lost their licenses and 66% were required to do some kind of education and/or supervision in order to continue their practice.

Creating an analogy from these percentages, we find:

From a hypothetical 1000 therapists over a 6 year period
110 of these 1000 therapists would be "grieved"
25 of these 1000 would have their cases investigated
14 of these 1000 would be "found against"
9 of these 1000 would be given remedial education and/or supervision requirements
5 of these 1000 would lose their license to practice

Another set of statistics from 2005[xlv] reveals similar results.

Total Active Licenses/Registrations .... = 60,766
Complaints Received .... = 1,010
Suspension or Surrender of License .... = 13
%age of Total Active licensed clinicians grieved..... = 1.7%
%age of Total Active licensed clinicians whose licenses
*   were suspended or surrendered............. . = .02%*

For psychologists, reports Ofer Zur, "less than 2% faced any licensing complaints between 1996 and 2000. Not all complaints are investigated, and of those that are, 30 percent are determined not to be in violation. All in all, less than 0.4 percent of psychologists have faced any reportable action by licensing boards.   The percentage of complaints against counselors and social workers is even lower."[xlvi]

Extrapolating these statistics gives a more realistic picture of therapists who are grieved. Understand that the Grievance Board is there both for the protection of clients from harm and for the protection of mental health practitioners from false accusations. It is clear that the vast majority of therapists use their power ethically. It is also true that these cases do not represent all the harm experienced by clients (and sometimes therapists). Additional ethical violations are *never* reported because the violations were resolved in other ways. Some were not reported or resolved due to the client's lack of knowledge, fear or disempowerment, e.g. not knowing that a therapist's behavior was unethical, not knowing there is a grievance procedure, taking personal responsibility for the difficulty, or thinking that the harm wasn't serious enough to warrant reporting it.

What are some actual grievance cases and what were the rulings?

On the next page are examples of Grievances and Disciplinary Actions of the Colorado Mental Health Boards[xlvii] between March 1, 2001 and February 28, 2002. All of these were cases in which the therapist was "found against" in an investigation.

Grievance	Board Action
Sexual contact with a client; maintained an inappropriate relationship with client; provided services that fall below generally accepted standards of practice	Injunction to prohibit/restrain practice
Substance abuse relapse (self-report)	1 year Stipulation for restricted practice
Failed to keep essential client records within generally-accepted standards of practice	Letter of Admonition
Provided services outside area of training or competence; failed to consult or refer a client to an appropriate practitioner	Revocation of CAC (Addiction Counselor) Certification
Breached client confidentiality	Letter of Admonition
Convicted of sexual assault on a child by a person in a position of trust	Revocation of License
Provided services outside area of training, experience or competence; maintained a dual relationship with a client; failed to consult; failed to refer	Revocation of License

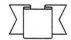

Felony conviction which effects ability to practice	Injunction to prohibit/restrain practice
Failed to report child abuse when it was reasonable, prudent, and necessary to do so	Letter of Admonition
Misrepresented credentials	Letter of Admonition

Another sample of unethical behaviors heard in Grievance Hearings in the State of Colorado (without listing of ruling):

- A counselor who diagnosed every client as a victim of ritual abuse.
- A male psychiatrist who told each of his female clients that they were very special, that this had never happened before, and that he had fallen in love with them. Then he initiated sexual contact.
- A therapist who advertised as a doctor and had false Ph.D. diplomas on his wall.
- A Social Worker who frequently lost her temper with clients and with other professional colleagues.
- A therapist who consistently convinced clients that they needed more and more therapy.

The following is a record of complaints phoned in to a bodywork Ethics Committee (from Sept 1996 to Sept 1998). Note: no information is included about what kind of action was taken or which complaints were dismissed, resolved or withdrawn. Complaint:

- Body work produced no change
- Client was dropped by practitioner with no explanation
- Practitioner dropped client because practitioner thought Bodywork wasn't helping, but client did feel it was helping and wanted to continue
- Practitioner made sexual advances toward client
- Practitioner engaged in inappropriate hugging
- Practitioner asked questions that were too intimate
- Practitioner didn't address client's physical concern
- Client paid in advance for a series of sessions, when offered a price break and then wanted to stop before completing sessions and did not get the money back.

Note: Most of these appear to be relationship issues that the practitioner could have noticed and handled within the relationship.

Several examples from the California Board of Behavioral Sciences, Spring 2006 newsletter:

• Respondent began a therapeutic relationship with a client that lasted approximately 4-5 weeks. Respondent admitted terminating the therapeutic relationship in order to pursue an intimate and sexual relationship with the client.

• For approximately nine months, respondent engaged in a professional therapeutic relationship with a patient whom she diagnosed as suffering from Dissociative Identity Disorder....Respondent's 24-hour DID training....did not satisfactorily prepare her to adequately treat a patient with DID. Respondent allowed extreme levels of counter-transference to override sound clinical decisions....thereby compromising the health and safety of the patient who was suicidal. Respondent created a dual relationship, including a close personal relationship with a patient that was emotionally and physically predatory and clinically unsafe, thereby.... exposing the client to the risk of emotional harm.

What kinds of issues do psychologists find most ethically troubling?

In an interesting study reported in Kenneth Pope and Valerie Vetter asked a random sample of members of the APA to "describe incidents that they found ethically challenging or troubling....679 psychologists described 703 incidents in 23 categories." I'll name some of these categories here. This kind of research is "useful in considering possible revisions of the code. . . . that address realistically the emerging dilemmas that confront us in the day-to-day work of psychology."[xlviii]

CATEGORY	PERCENT	NUMBER
Confidentiality	*18%*	*128*
Blurred, dual, or conflictual relationships	*17%*	*116*
Payment sources, plans, settings, and methods	*14%*	*97*
Academic settings, teaching dilemmas, & concerns	*8%*	*57*
Conduct of colleagues	*4%*	*29*
Sexual issues	*4%*	*28*
Assessment	*4%*	*25*
Questionable or harmful interventions	*3%*	*20*
Competence	*3%*	*20*
Helping the financially stricken	*2%*	*13*
Supervision	*2%*	*13*
Advertising and (mis)representation	*1%*	*13*
Termination	*1%*	*5*

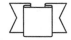

Ethnicity	1%	4
Treatment records	1%	4

xlix

Why do things go wrong?

"Ethics violations don't usually happen because someone does not know the rules. They happen because of some kind of internal misalignment with power." [1]

Using our power of communication, presence and position not only to prevent or reduce harm, but also to promote well-being, requires us to know our ourselves and our role differential. These are evolutions in personal and professional development recommended in Right Use of Power. For more about this question, please refer to Power Differential pages 29-30, Factors and Cognitive Strategies pages 89-91, Personal Power page 107-108, Shame page 115-116, Resolving Difficulties page 207-210, Grievance Processes page 225, Shadow aspects of increased power pages 303-306, and Power Paradox pages 316-319.

Some factors to consider

Accusations and rumors of unethical behavior tend to be shocking and black and white, engendering the twins of self-righteousness and shame. By being compassionate and realistic, we can understand why we in the helping professions sometimes use our power in unethical ways. Here are a few factors.

- Naïveté (either genuine not knowing the standard or not what you should know about right use of power)
- Relational clumsiness or awkwardness
- Thinking you can get away with it
- Self-protection and/or survival
- Silence, non-action, or aggression out of fear, shame, or embarrassment
- Counter-transference
- Poor judgment
- Greed
- Personal need for power and/or control
- Corrupted perception of power differential role
- Inability to be compassionate or empathic
- Pain

- Revenge
- Re-enactment
- Misplaced ego needs for love, power, respect, sex, money, intimacy
- Desperation
- Stress
- Inability to access social engagement nervous system

Cognitive Strategies

"When we feel threatened, communication gets distorted."
Peg Syverson

When we behave unethically, we often use cognitive strategies to justify our behavior. Pope and Vasquez have identified 21 of these "Ethical Fallacies." Here are a few of them. These are essentially ways that we fool ourselves into thinking that our behavior is actually not unethical. We find ways to think about a situation to justify it to ourselves and to others. As Pope and Vasquez put it, "All of us face the human temptation to duck important ethical responsibilities. Temptation grows stronger when we're tired, afraid, under pressure, or in conflict. . . . We believe that the overwhelming majority of psychologists are conscientious, caring individuals, committed to ethical behavior. We also believe that none of us is infallible and that perhaps all of us, at one time or another, have been vulnerable to at least a few of these ethical justifications."

"Sometime down the road at a moment of terrible need, temptation, exhaustion, carelessness, narcissism, anger, lack of perspective, or confusion, an ethical fallacy that once struck us as ridiculous may suddenly emerge as wise, profound, and practical."[ii]

Here are a few of them.
1) It's not unethical as long as a managed care administrator or insurance case reviewer required or suggested it.
3) It's not unethical if an ethics code never mentions the concept, term, or act.
4) It's not unethical as long as no law was broken.
6) It's not unethical as long as we can name others who do the same thing.
7) It's not unethical as long as we didn't mean to hurt anyone.

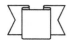

8) It's not unethical even if our acts have caused harm as the person we harmed had it coming, provoked us, deserved it, was really asking for it, or has not behaved perfectly.

10) It's not unethical if we could not (or did not) anticipate the unintended consequences of our acts.

12) It's not unethical if we can say any of the following about it (feel free to extend the list):

"What else could I do?"
"Anyone else would've done the same thing."
"It came from the heart."
"I listened to my soul."
"I went with my gut."
"I just knew that's what my client/student needed."
"I'd do the same thing again if I had it to do over."
"It worked before."
"I'm only human, you know!"
"What's the big deal?

17) It's not unethical as long as it results in a higher income or more prestige.

19) It's not unethical as long as it would be almost impossible to do things another way.

21) It's not unethical as long as we can find a consultant who says its OK. [lii]

These may seem ridiculous to read, but we are all vulnerable and we all get stressed, tempted, tired, and not at our best. Being aware of these cognitive fallacies can help us be pro-active in catching ourselves in flawed-thinking.

Compassion for the harm we cause others, no matter what the reasons, is a challenging endeavor. The Dalai Lama, when asked about the definition of compassion, described a man beating a dog. Compassion, he said, is when you feel as much for the man as for the dog. *"Unresolved emotional pain is the great contagion of our time—of all time. This does not deny the struggle for justice: There IS a world out there, and it cries out for rectification. But those who cannot sense the pain of the one who wounds them will dispense, under the banner of righteousness, a misshapen justice, and create yet more enduring wrongs."* [liii]

Good judgment comes from experience. Experience comes from bad judgment.   *—Barry LePatner[liv]*

Compassion Practice: Take three breaths.   *—CB*

Self-study practice: Walking in other moccasins

When you treat yourself with compassion, your aspirations will stretch you in the direction of increasingly better ethical behavior. Compassion begins at home with yourself. The more self-awareness, compassion, willingness to take responsibility for your behavior, freedom from shame, and ability to tell the truth about yourself, the easier it will be for you to act with moral integrity.

Please find the place inside you that knows how to be compassionate. Now extend that compassion through your body and your space. Offer yourself some compassion. Now extend this compassion into the room, the community, the world and beyond. Still continuing to feel your compassion, take a few minutes to remember an unethical behavior that you know about. Now imagine what might have been going on for the person who behaved unethically. Send compassion to that person.

Take some time and then return to ordinary consciousness. Use the chart on the next page to summarize your responses.

1. Unethical behavior(s)
2. Specific Grievance(s)

3. Imagined cause(s)
4. Recommendations for a. remediation   b. re-education

Example:
1. Unethical behavior: explosiveness, poor decision-making, absences, emotional ups and downs due to addiction to pain killers.
2. Specific grievance(s): services failed to meet generally accepted standards, impaired judgment).
3. Cause: self-protection and/or survival, poor judgment, desperation, stress.
4. Recommendation for remediation: removal from position until addiction has been handled. Recommendation for re-education: personal work to handle stress better.

Dimension Two:
Be Compassionate and Aware

Topics covered in this section:
Personal Power
Shame
Non-ordinary States
Touch
Sexuality
Transference

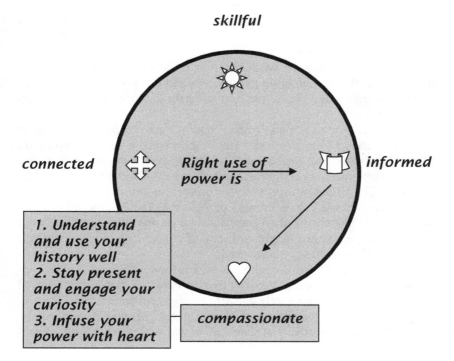

skillful

connected   *Right use of* ⟶   *informed*
                           power is

compassionate

1. **Understand and use your history well**
2. **Stay present and engage your curiosity**
3. **Infuse your power with heart**

Focus on Awareness

- *Right Use of Power is being conscious about your impact.*
- *Dimension Two is about Awareness.*

    - *Being curious about and tracking how your use of power affects your clients*

    - *Understanding and using your history in relation to issues of power and authority*

    - *Engaging your compassion*

    - *Exploring a range of qualities of power*

    - *Understanding how shame limits awareness and responsiveness*

    - *Noticing how non-ordinary states of consciousness increase vulnerability*

Power Spiral—Topics in the Awareness Dimension

The diagram places the conscious use of power at the bottom of the power spiral. This is directionally in the South. The focus is on Self[iv] and there are three skills and wisdoms. These are: to be curious, to understand and use your history, and to engage your curiosity. Topical material covers the following information:

•   We learn about the wisdom of our profession through the written ethics codes. We pay attention to ourselves and our personal history with power and authority. We reflect on our habits, tendencies and beliefs around power.

•   We engage in self-study about how we use our personal power in order to increase our awareness and responsiveness to our impact on others. We think about themes such as: What about your power concerns you? In what situations do you dis-empower yourself and how do you do this? What is the shadow aspect of your power and how does it emerge?

•   We increase our awareness of power of the heightened state of consciousness that clients often enter during a session. When in this altered state, clients are also in a heightened state of sensitivity and as a result will be more easily and strongly influenced.

•   We look at the complex, sensitive, and challenging topics of sexuality and therapeutic use of touch. How to hold clear sexual boundaries and use touch safely and effectively is covered.

•   We address the feeling of shame and its history, dynamics, and impact. We study the effects of shame as an ethical issue that compromises consciousness and connection. We understand the often surprising power of transference in professional relationships, as it is linked with the power differential.

Three Skills and Wisdoms
Understand and use your history well
Curiosity quiets judgment and/or blame. It lightens the heart and opens natural pathways to healing and well-being. Curiosity is disarming, spacious, and contagious.

We all have dynamic relationships with our power. By uncovering our beliefs and habits around issues of power, authority, and influence, we are more able to use power skillfully and benevolently; free of misguided beliefs and compensations.

Stay present and engage your curiosity
Truly showing up and being sensitive, open and flexible with those who are in down-power roles while at the same time staying in charge in the ways that are needed by the role sets the foundation for right relationship.

Infuse your power with heart
Compassion is the feeling through which we gain access to the felt sense of others as different but not separate. Curiosity and empathy are two valuable keys to right relationship with power. They are connecting links between power and heart.

Barriers and Resources
Becoming more sensitive and aware in the use of your personal and role power may involve learning about the barriers and resources that either block or help your awareness of your power. **Barriers to awareness** seem to be stimulated by shame or fear of being overwhelmed by the pain of remembering old wounds of power. Habits that interfere with awareness include: numbing, disconnecting from the heart, and discounting experience. We study limiting beliefs such as "If I remember, I'll never stop crying." "I was so hurt, I decided I'd never risk being powerful and maybe hurting someone else." "I need to protect people from my power." "No one will get to me again."

In telling stories and working with the exercises and topics in this section, participants have gained insights such as: "Power is a feedback loop for self-knowledge." "I can be humble in my power." "I have a feeling in my bones that I don't have to be ashamed, ambivalent, or hide my power anymore." "I'm ready to claim my history differently."

Resources for awareness include recognizing the golden thread of our woundedness, increasing tracking skills, and de-activating shame.

Power Spiral Layer

The layer of the Power Spiral associated with the South dimension describes the four focuses of the Right Use of Power. The focus for each dimension is related to the same dimension in other rings of the spiral. After focusing on information in Dimension One, the focus shifts to self-awareness in Dimension Two. Relationship is the focus of Dimension Three, and Wisdom the focus of Dimension Four.

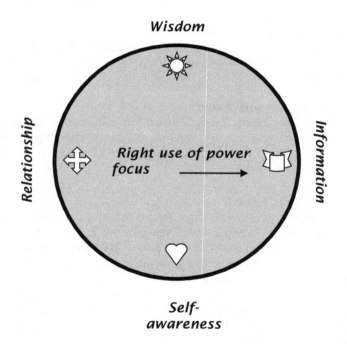

Being Informed

This is surely the information age. Accuracy and engagement with information leads directly to understanding our empowered and disempowered Selves and to greater confidence. Relationships are clearer, and cleaner when we approach them with self-knowledge. Wisdom is the result of being well-informed, self-aware, and compassionately related.

Personal Power

Story: *Robert's client Henry complained of tightness and pain in his lower back and thighs. He spoke of constantly and actively being on guard for danger so that he could be ready to take protective action. Robert asked Henry to show him how he guarded. Henry described having power in his fingertips that could send out flashes of lightning if anyone threatened. His eyes surveyed and he held his chest up. His whole body was taut with readiness to assert his power. Robert asked about what the alertness was protecting. Henry replied, "My heart." Robert asked Henry to take his awareness from his fingers to his heart and belly and notice what he experienced. After a long silence, Henry spoke. "I see that when I bring my power and awareness back to my belly, I feel quite strong and safe. When I have my power out in my fingertips, I scare people and isolate myself. And, to my surprise, I feel desperate and much <u>less</u> powerful. You know, like 'more bark than bite'. After another silence, Henry noticed that his lower back was relaxing. The pain was connected to putting his power outside rather than inside.*

Take a minute to notice what your experience of the word "power" is . . . .Generally, most initial and automatic responses to the word power include concepts like forceful, controlling, manipulative, insensitive, violent, hurtful, invulnerable. Power seems to be most often conceptualized in a monolithic way, based on power as strength. This conception causes harm when power-as-strength is used to dominate or manipulate. As a psychotherapist put it, "*My response to hearing the word was negative, reflecting my feelings of fear associated with power. I don't like conflict and so I give away my personal power and compromise my true feelings to maintain peace. As I reflected further, I became aware of an old belief that if I am too powerful, the person may disagree with me, create conflict, and then dislike me. This is something I would like to change. I want to claim my personal power.*"

Students' drawings of their history in relation to power are predominantly traumatic or painful ones and are most often related to childhood experiences with parents, teachers, or religious leaders. One caregiver drew a picture of her experience of being abused as a child and then folded and folded her picture into a tiny wad that she colored red.

This wad poignantly symbolized her childhood (and now adult) response to this misuse of power—wadding herself up as small as possible to protect herself. She then asked the group to support her in unfolding herself by touching the wad of paper. As she passed the red picture around, others tearfully acknowledged their own experiences of making themselves small or making themselves too big. The caregiver then, disengaging from her shame, slowly and deliberately unfolded her drawing, re-owning her power. The intensity of the moment was punctuated by her laughter, "Watch out! Instead of being a low maintenance person, I might become a medium maintenance person!" Drawings like this one represent the woundings of power that was used to rigidly control behavior and punish misbehavior by shaming. Modeling of benevolent uses of power is much needed to repair these woundings. A student said, *"What I have been taught about power presents a model I don't want to replicate. I need to transform power into a useful tool rather than something to be wary or frightened of. Then I can reinvent my approach to power and use it in a positive way."*

Redefining Power and Influence

Power is neutral. Power is the capacity to bring change. It is, of course, how we use our power and influence that makes all the difference. Our most advanced methodologies and technologies are benevolent when used with an ethic of power just as evolved, formulated, and researched.

The Right Use of Power differs from familiar images of power in that the focus of attention is toward staying in right relationship. As one student says, *"Focusing on the issue of power—how I use it, how I feel about my own and about others'—awakens this issue and gives me the language and tools to explore it."*

Looking at power as relational and benevolent, there are a number of aspects to examine.

Bringing dreams to fruition

Personal power is needed in the creative process of bringing your dreams to fruition, in making real your intentions, in manifesting your gifts, in embodying your aspirations. As Starhawk says,

"The root of power means to be able. Power from within is linked to the mysteries that awaken our deepest abilities and potential. So if our work is to evoke power-from-within, we must clearly envision the conditions that would allow that power to come forth. We must identify

what blocks it, and create the conditions that foster empowerment. Given a
world based on power-over, we must remake the world."[lvi]

The source of your power

Seeking power, we must tend to the inner source, as if tilling the soil
of the Self. What do you think of as the source of your power? There are
many levels to this question. There is the kind of power that automatically
accompanies your role as a helping professional. There is the
body/mind/spirit power that provides the concrete ability to act or have
influence. And there is the more elusive level of ultimate source. Some
believe that this is God and that all they do is a result of God acting
through them; some believe that they are channeling a higher power or
resonating "field" of energy and information; some believe that personal
power is an evolution of human consciousness. Most of us seem to have
some sense that there is a power larger than Self that we are guided by or
in collaboration with. Whatever your belief, there may be a shadow side in
which this source of power, however you refer to it, could be exploited or
misunderstood, or used with undue influence, e.g. *"This message for you
came to me from God; My inner guidance is always trustworthy; This
suffering is his karma; or The higher power has something special in
mind; or God is on our side."* Whatever your belief, it is important to name
and acknowledge your experience of source and to watch out for misuses
of this source.

Cultural messages about power

A wide range of cultural messages about power influences your beliefs
about power, your responses to power, and your use of your power. Most
of these are unconscious until you identify and explore them. The
following are examples of common influences: your gender, race, ethnic
background, body size and shape, religious preference, class, age, sexual
preference, disabilities, military experience, English as second language,
status as an immigrant, extended family, primary decision-maker/head of
household, and involvement in groups or clubs. A significant part of
understanding how you use your power comes from identifying the
messages about power that are part of your personal and cultural history.

Qualities of power

Strength, control, and force are the most common qualities associated
with power. The power to create and influence actually comes through
many additional qualities, such as kindness, collaboration, yielding,

spaciousness, and enthusiasm. Research done by Angeles Arrien[lvii] describes three kinds of power commonly recognized by native peoples throughout the world. These three kinds of power provide a broader lens for understanding power.

• *Power of position* refers to the ability to influence through role and authority, i.e., through conscious use of the power differential. Those skilled in the power of position use their role to maintain safety, protect their client's spirit, take responsibility for relationship health, empower their clients, and see a wider perspective. The Hakomi Institute Code of Ethics[lviii] puts it this way: *"The impact of the role-based power difference between client and therapist is very strong and also very subtle, and thus demands a strong ethical stance."*

• *Power of presence* is an under-acknowledged power. Power of presence is the capacity to influence through your personhood, wisdom, attention, and being in the moment. Those skilled in the power of presence create an atmosphere of safety, warmth, compassion and respect. Difficulties seldom arise and when they do, they are attended to without delay or escalation.

• *Power of communication* is the ability to have an effect through speaking and writing clearly, verbalizing empathy, managing and focusing important and meaningful information, encouraging dialogue, and inspiring and galvanizing others to take action. Those skilled in the power of communication take charge when needed, perceive and effectively convey vital information, listen well, and communicate clearly and concisely. They know how and when to repair and self-correct.

Wise healing and teaching work engages all three kinds of power. Many studies show that the power of presence, the ability of the therapist to create a safe and healing relationship, is, in fact, more important than the particular therapeutic modality that is used.

Dynamic and magnetic qualities

Dynamic power is active, charismatic, directing, informing, diagnosing, and discriminating. Magnetic power works through receptivity, inclusiveness, attention to the atmosphere, collaboration, spaciousness, flexibility, and modeling. (Dynamic and magnetic are more inclusive and less charged words for active and passive or masculine and feminine.) Both are effective, but they are experienced differently and represent differing models of leadership. The most effective leaders are able to use both and each at the right time.

Uses of Power in the Four Dimensions

Four kinds of power align with the four dimensions of the power spiral.

1. The power of **information**. Your power expresses through your ability to integrate and communicate ideas, insights, and understandings.

2. The power of **Self**. Your power expresses through your personhood and your ability to be centered, and charismatic.

3. The power of **connectedness**. Your power expresses through your ability to be in right relationship and to understand systems and their dynamics.

4. The power of **vision**. Your power expresses through your ability to see the whole and future possibilities and from this vision inspire and create.

These qualities are further described in the chapter on Leadership.

Power Parameters

We tend to think of and respond to power as if it had one basic quality: force. However, when understanding power as the ability to have an effect or to have influence, the number of ways to have this influence increases dramatically. Here is a chart that names just a few power parameters. Each of these has a continuum for its use.

To create a little picture of yourself in relation to how you use your power, place yourself with a mark somewhere along each of the following continuums. In the use of your power, where along the continuum from one extreme to another do you tend to land? As you go through this list, you will probably notice that it is difficult to select a spot because where you put your mark varies by the situation. This is a good thing. You want to have the ability to stretch along the healthy parameters of these continuums to respond appropriately. However, most people can identify a spot on each line that is a general tendency. You might want to put different colored marks along the lines to indicate your tendencies in the following situations: general, in up-power roles, in down-power roles and with friends and family. Are there major differences or are they minor? What do you make of this? Notice which continuums are marked closest to the extremes? These are qualities you might want to be especially watchful about to prevent harm. Try out stretching your healthy range a bit. How do you imagine your relationships would change if you had a wider range?

Some Power Parameters

directive ————————————— **responsive**
(dynamic, controlling)   *(magnetic, adaptive)*

firm ——————————————— **flexible**
(invulnerable, boundaried)   *(vulnerable, unboundaried)*

task focused —————— **relationship focused**
(structured)   *(unstructured)*

persist——————————————**let go**
(maintain, hold on)   *(surrender, delay)*

truth-focused —————— **harmony-focused**

strength-centered —————— **heart-centered**

extroverted —————— **introverted**

(left margin, vertical: misuses of power at extremes)
(right margin, vertical: misuses of power at extremes)

In going through the above list, you probably noticed that all the qualities are necessary functions in the wise use of power. However, misuses of power tend to happen when someone is operating at either extreme of each continuum. For example, someone who is always very directive may cause harm by force or manipulation. Someone who always surrenders may cause harm by not taking charge. You may also notice that at either extreme, people get isolated and disconnected from relationship. For example, when someone is extremely truth-focused, the person and the caring relationship get lost.   When someone is extremely harmony-focused, real and important relationship differences and challenges get lost.   Maturity, satisfaction, and skillfulness depend on your ability to differentiate and integrate the skills on both sides of each continuum. The ability to use each skill when needed is essential to refining the art of Right Use of Power. We can be more effective when we can discern:

- when to take action and when to delay taking action;
- when to take charge and when to be flexible;
- when to focus on a task and when to focus on relationship maintenance.

My husband, Reynold Feldman, and I found the information connected with these parameters to be so valuable that we wrote a book whose central theme is that most misuses and abuses of personal and role power happen at behavioral extremes where people disconnect from both self and others. Find this book, *Living in the Power Zone,* at www.rightuseofpower.org.

Managing Polarities

A further refinement of working with these functions and tendencies is through looking at them as polarities to be harmonized. Barry Johnson[lix] has developed a process for working with polarities that's very helpful. The image he uses is an infinity sign.

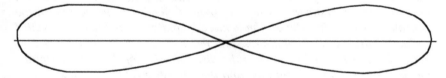

In the infinity symbol, as related to polarities, find your habitual and most comfortable place along the linear continuums between extremes. Know that in the natural, organic process of everyday life, we encounter polarities. Balancing polarities is one of the most basic life sustaining and creating processes. In the very simplest understanding of chaos theory,[lx] life can exist only in a fairly narrow band in which there's enough chaos to respond to new situations creatively and flexibly and yet not so much chaos that life becomes unmanageable. Viewed from the opposite polarity, to have enough order to maintain identity, but not so much order that adaptability is impossible.

Within this life sustaining band, there is constant movement toward the edge, self-correcting, balancing and rebalancing. It is not possible or life-enhancing to find the "perfect balanced position" and stay there. Living with the polarities is a dynamic and extraordinary process that enables the wonder and magic of creative resolution. Polarities create complex systems, and these exist within the complexities of power dynamics.

Working with polarities begins by walking the infinity sign (literally or figuratively) and getting in touch with the way that healthy and resilient living systems can quite naturally self-correct and regain their balance.

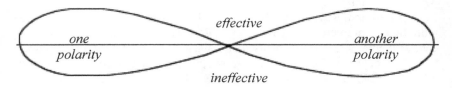

In order to work with the polarity system, start anywhere on the infinity symbol, move toward one polarity until it becomes ineffective and takes you down into the ineffective realm. Then begin to self-correct and move back toward the other polarity until *it* becomes ineffective. Then begin to self-correct and move the other way again.

Here's an example: *My most comfortable teaching style is spacious and flexible. When I get too spacious and flexible, my students get lost and have trouble understanding where to focus (effective to ineffective in the spaciousness polarity). When I'm centered, confident, and tracking well, I can notice the signs of imbalance, and move toward being more directive and ordered. I then move toward the directive side of the polarity until I notice signs of too much rigidity, and then move to rebalance in the other direction. The main three indicators of imbalance for me are: Students are confused. I'm not sure what is needed next. I experience an anxious feeling that people aren't getting what they need. Three strategies for re-balancing are: take a break, focus toward a specific topic, remind myself that when I'm direct, people* **will** *find their places.*

"Being in the flow" is the exciting and nourishing process of effortlessly using power to balance and rebalance. Like sailing a sailboat to a point on another shore, we don't get there by going straight ahead, but by making constant little or big adjustments. Letting go of finding the perfect solution we can accept balancing as an important function in creating and sustaining. Compassionately living polarities is both the goal and the process.

There are three ways to manage the polarities with ease.

1. Accept that balancing and adjusting is a natural and healthy process.

2. Make your infinity movement smaller. The less extreme the polarity, the easier it is to re-balance. Extremes have great learning, excitement, and growth value. Balancing them creates harmony.

3. Increase your sensitivity to signs of ineffectiveness and find effective strategies for re-balancing.

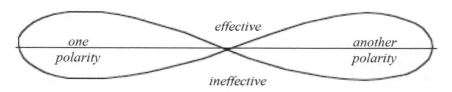

Indicators of Imbalance	*Strategies for Rebalance*

Understanding your history

To be able to use your history, you must know your history. Your personal history is a combination of your personal and cultural experiences with power, your beliefs about what power is and how it works, and your strategies for using or avoiding power. Personal understanding will help you avoid unconsciously repeating the kind of harm that you experienced and will help you be compassionate toward yourself and others.

Many people who choose the helping professions do so, at least in part, to heal their own past. They may want to make a difference in the world, or to not repeat the woundings that they experienced from people who misused their power. To avoid causing more harm, helping professionals may tend to avoid using power, under-use power, or withdraw from it.. Right Use of Power ethics work is focused toward re-owning and honoring power as the ability to have good effect.

Power of stories

Stories are powerful tools for healing and understanding. And our own stories are vehicles for healing and understanding. We can't change the past, but we can learn from it. We can reconsider the decisions and strategies we made from past experience, and we can discover the golden thread. Uncovering the ways we may have over-compensated can prevent unwitting harm or confusion for our clients, colleagues and friends. Stories are non-blaming and non-judgmental ways to impart difficult learnings.

This particular story influenced the way I respond to my clients. *Many years ago, when I was in my 20s, I was in a therapy group, consciously practicing being direct about my feelings and responses to others in the group. I felt upset and angry about something the group leader said and told her that I felt angry with her. She responded by saying, "Well, let's look at how this is connected to your relationship with your mother.* I answered this set of questions about this memory that helped me understand the impact and update some of my beliefs.

1. What is your experience? *Feeling discounted, put down, embarrassed, withdrawing.*	2. What was the impact on the relationship? *Loss of trust. Left the group.*
3. What would you have needed from the person who hurt you in order for this to have turned out okay? *I needed her to accept responsibility for her impact, offer to work on improving our relationship, and acknowledge by courage and caring. I needed her to demonstrate being an authentic and vulnerable person.*	4. What decisions about power did you make as a result of this event? *Interactions should be taken personally. There is some germ of any feedback that is personal. To earn trust, leaders must be real in their role power. I decided I would never dismiss a client or student's feedback.*
5. How else has this experience shaped you? *I am sensitive to how authentic and real leaders are.*	6. What did the person who hurt you NOT know? *She didn't understand the effect of the power differential in making it very difficult for clients to offer critical feedback. She didn't know how to respond non-defensively, and she didn't know that every client response isn't a projection.*
7. What did you learn from this experience? (your "golden thread") *Increased sensitivity to feedback as a combination of personal and projection. High priority on being real and accessible as a teacher/therapist while still holding the boundaries of my role.*	8. Have you over-compensated in any way was a result of this experience? How? *I take feedback too personally without including context, and the personal history of the student/client, and habitual responses to leadership role.*

To help illuminate this process a bit more, here are some additional examples from students:

What did you decide about power based on this incident?

> *"Power gets in the way of belonging."*
>
> *"Power is cruel, oppressive, and bad. So I'm not going to use it."*
>
> *"Silence is power, therefore, I'll just be quiet from now on."*

These are decisions that turned into beliefs that turned into habits, ones that cause harm to self and others and interfere with the person's ability to use their power wisely and well. How relieving and transformative it is to understand the belief, where it came from and how it is affecting life and work in the present! With this knowledge comes the ability to update the old belief to a new one that will serve better.

Summary

Personal power is a complex and dynamic set of tendencies, beliefs, polarities, and preferences. Rather than simply being equated with strength, Right Use of Power calls for a broad understanding of the many qualities and energies that power comprises in its richest spectrum. Personal power, understood and developed, is the strong foundation for being able to use role power wisely and effectively. Personal power is dynamic, accessible and unique. It may be impacted by others, but belongs to Self. Personal power, as the core of Self, is independent of the opinions of others.

Personal power expresses itself in relationships. Marc Barasch[lxi] offers his wisdom: *"Unless we are solitary anchorites, cartoon hermits with beards grown down to our toes, we live in relationship, which guarantees we will be hurt by others and inevitably will hurt them...To accept our own hurt, taking it in rather than projecting it out, distills the healing elixir."*[lxii] Healing itself is a product of patience, the passage of time, the appropriate expression of anger, compassion or forgiveness, and ultimately personal choice.

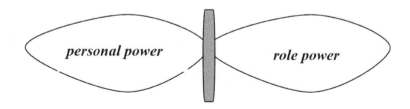

personal power   *role power*

Like having two wings, we can fly with both personal and role power in balance.

Mastery in the use of your power for good is a lifetime process. Self-study makes it easier to use your history to advantage. A massage therapist reflected, *"If someone had said to me 15 years ago, after having been so wounded by sexual abuse, that I would today be using my hands in the gift of healing, I would have said, 'How is that possible?'" I would have been bound by fear. But the power of grace is that often there is a gift in the wound that can open into the very gift we are to bring to others."*

Stepping Into My Power
Marie McCagno

Stepping into my power
Feels like crossing
a glacier-fed stream.
Fast-flowing water pushing
at my calves, shins, ankles
As I brace my feet,
Finding my ground,
supported by a rocky creek bed.
Before my next move
I pause, breathe, choose;
Believing in the moment
This is possible, while
Numbingly cold water
makes my feet ache
My attention focused
on the here and now
Of each move.
Stepping into my power
means
Finding my voice
Hearing my words take
flight,
making space.
Feeling my knowing
deep in my belly
Feeds my connections.

Alive and aware

Self-study Practices

1. Cultural Messages

Take a minute now to identify a few messages about power that come from your cultural background. Pick one or more and respond to items A - D.

CULTURE	MESSAGE
• Class • Sex • Nationality • Race • Age • Education • Employment	A. MESSAGE received about power. B. HOW does this message effect how I use my personal and/or role power? C. Have these messages caused me to feel DISEMPOWERED? D. What are some NEW WAYS OF THINKING, FEELING, OR BEHAVING that might help me mediate the impact of these beliefs and make me feel more powerful?
Sex: Female	One person's responses: A."I received the message that women should stay in the background and support men, so B. I'm reluctant to take charge or be directive when I'm in an up-power position. C. Obviously, I feel disempowered most of the time when in the company of men. D. I can understand that this is a cultural, not factual, belief and begin experimenting with putting myself forward more and learning to discern what situations will be most supportive of my new behavior."

2. Reflecting on your history

This self-study process offers you an opportunity to explore your humanness in an experiential way and then share your story if you choose. Get comfortable; breathe, relax, close your eyes, and turn your awareness to your inside world. From your inward awareness notice your experience of yourself right now. You might notice your thoughts, sensations, breathing, emotions, images—any or all of these. Engage your curiosity and your compassion. We've all been hurt. Suffering is a universal human experience. You are not alone in it.

From a receptive place, please let your unconscious offer you a memory of a time when power was misused toward you by someone in a parental or professional relationship with you. Let this be a memory that is not too overwhelming—one that is still unresolved but available for further exploration and healing. This memory could be about anyone in a up-power position such as doctor, therapist, clergy, or a parent. . . .As you explore this memory, consider these questions.

1. What happened?	2. What was the impact on this relationship?
3. What would you have needed from the person who hurt you (that you didn't get) that would have made things turn out okay?	4. What decision(s) about power and about your power did you make as a result of this event?
5. How else did this incident shape you?	6. What did the person who hurt you NOT know? (Make a guess.)
7. What did you learn from this experience? (your golden thread)	8. Have you over-compensated in any way as a result of this experience? How?

Take your time, and when you have enough information, please let go of the memory and bring your attention back outward. Take a few moments to journal or draw. Then fill in the empty grid with your experience of the meditation.

One of my students, Rocio, realized something significant: *"It's not something that's wrong with me. It's something that happened to me."*[lxiii]

3. Walking the Map

Pick one of the power parameters listed on page 104 and explore how you walk this one on the infinity map.

- Name three familiar indicators of imbalance.

- Identify three specific behavioral strategies for getting back in balance.

- Referring to the parameters, what kinds of power challenges do you face in your habits and tendencies? What kinds of misuses of power might you make? What could you be especially alert about?

4. Compassion Practice

From the misuse of power experience you brought to mind in self-study 2, reflect on the question: What did the person who hurt you NOT know? Being compassionate and creative: If you could design a course for this person, what would be in the curriculum that could serve him or her to understand, self-correct, and use his or her power with more heart, wisdom and skill?

Shame

A psychology teacher asked her ethics class, "All of you agree with the rule about no dual relationships, right?" (All heads nodded.) Then he said, "So, let's get real here. I won't report this, but I'm curious. How many of you have had a dual relationship with a client? How many of you have betrayed confidentiality? How many of you have had to deal with feeling attracted to a client?" Most hands go up. "How many of you have ever talked with someone about any of these things?" One hand goes up. "Why not?" The overwhelming response: shame."

"Awareness of shame is one of the last great secrets, and it's not out yet,"[lxiv] says Dr. Terry Keepers. *"For reasons rooted in the values of contemporary culture, the concept of shame... has all but vanished from discussions of emotional disarray, instead of being regarded as the pre-eminent cause of emotional distress in our time. Because of its aversiveness, we go to great lengths to avoid it, thus creating serious denial, projection, isolation, and deeply guarded secrets,"* writes Robert Karen[lxv] in further support of the importance of addressing shame.

Shame is defined as a deeply disturbing, painful and irredeemable feeling of badness, disgrace, incompetence, unloveableness, indecency, or blame-worthiness. Shame is experienced as a global attack on the core Self that sentences the person to life with an irreparable flaw or inadequacy. Now considered a primary though under-acknowledged emotion, shame creates self-loathing or other-loathing and sometimes imploding or exploding rage. Remarkably, virtually everyone experiences shame. The feeling of shame comes in a wide range of severity.

Where does shame come from? There are many triggers. Here are a few--facial expression, advertising, religious doctrine, cultural messages, not fitting into a cultural norm, whispers or secrets, shunning, or comments or behavior of family members, teachers, clergy or others in up-power roles.

Shame is an ethics and power issue because it severely interferes with a practitioner's ability to recognize and take responsibility for actions or behaviors that have caused harm. Feeling shame therefore impedes the process of resolution and self-correction.

Accusations of unethical behavior, whether accurate or not, are often accompanied by exaggeration, shock, self-righteousness, outrage, and/or desire for revenge or severe punishment. Perhaps self-righteousness asserts itself because we want to keep the secret that we too feel ashamed.

When errors or mistakes are kept in secret shame, there is little possibility of repairing harm, acting accountably, and self-correcting. Situations then needlessly escalate and practitioners develop patterns of repeating the same misuses of power. By keeping it secret, we become stuck in shame.

Fear of shaming (or being shamed) is one reason colleagues tend to avoid talking directly with other colleagues about suspected misuses of power. Shame on the part of caregivers can result in defensiveness, denial, dissociation, rigidity, and fear of getting help or supervision.

The nature of the legal process, unfortunately, often supports lack of truthfulness, since legal proceedings focus on determining and punishing one guilty party rather than seeing who was harmed, how they were harmed, and what kind of repair is needed.

Some methods of teaching ethics over-focus on a small percentage of egregious ethical violations and the severity of grievance and legal procedures. This focus can be experienced as shaming and can engender ethics paranoia resulting in hyper-vigilance, rule-bound rigidity, and denial or avoidance, all of which further perpetuate shame. This is a self-reinforcing cycle.

The Influence of Shame

A shame experience inherently creates an inability to accurately reality check, disconnection from relationship, and, usually, denial. This makes it particularly difficult for practitioners to be accountable for their behavior. In fact, just being in an up-power role, can bring about shame. For example, a shame-related fear of incompetence.

My colleague, Morgan Holford[lxvi], speaks of these shame dynamics directly and succinctly:

- *When in shame, it is impossible to be fully and truly accountable.*

- *Accountability requires an accurate self-assessment and this is not possible because shame's self-assessment is of exaggerated, one-sided, negative, irreparable culpability.*

- *Accountability requires being in relationship with whomever has been injured or affected by one's actions. When in shame, one is disconnected in withdrawal or anger.*

- *Accountability requires a groundedness and openness that are extremely difficult when in shame because one's tendency is to defend, focus on good intentions, disregard impact, and get lost in feelings.*

A student's insight: *"Until I can be accountable for the wrong actions I have taken, or even for the negative impact of actions that weren't necessarily wrong, healing and relationship repair cannot happen."*

Shame and the human nervous system

It is clear that shame interferes with interpersonal relatedness. Stephen Porges[lxvii] explains why. His theory has been summarized here by Inge Mula Myllerup.[lxviii] Humans and other mammals may be viewed as having three levels of nervous system activation: The first level is the level of activation which Steven Porges has named 'the social engagement nervous system.' This system is activated when a mammal, human or other, is interacting with another and connecting with eye contact and with verbal and/or non-verbal affective interaction without overwhelming experiences of fear. The second level of nervous system activation kicks in if and when a mammal perceives a situation as dangerous. The nervous system responds with sympathetic hyper-arousal. A flight/fight reaction is triggered with physiological activation of muscles in the arms and legs, leading the mammal to be inclined to either run to get away, or when this is not possible, to fight their way out of a situation. The third level of nervous system activation is a sympathetic hypo-arousal. This reaction kicks in when a mammal experiences a situation as life threatening without possibility for escape. The mammal freezes, arms and legs go limp and there is a dimming of life force. The mammal essentially plays dead. The three levels are listed schematically below.

concern	danger	life threat
social engagement	*hit/run*	*freeze*

When someone experiences shame (depending on the intensity of psychological resourcefulness of the person), this feeling may take them directly to the most primal nervous system response—the freeze response. This level and intensity of shame may be a perceived threat to Self and thus to survival. When in freeze response, it is impossible to connect and resource. When helping someone return to social engagement, it is useful to bridge through the three levels of nervous system activation. This means first helping the person activate by moving their arms and legs and turning their head to re-orient, and then helping them get back into social engagement through touch, sound, and eye contact.

Self-Study Practice: Recognizing Shame

Gather some paper and colors and then get comfortable. Turn your awareness inside. Now invite your unconscious to offer you a not-so-charged memory of a time when you felt shame. Tune in to your felt sense—your body, spirit, mind, sensations, posture. . . . . Don't stay in the memory long, but just enough time for a taste. Then bring your attention back. Get up and move or stretch, and then take some time to draw or write about your experience. When you have gathered your perceptions, express them in a drawing. Spend a little time with your drawing. How are you affected? What have you discovered? What triggered your shame event? What does the shame need?

These are common physiological descriptions in response to shame. *How do they compare to your experience? Do you relate to any of these experiences in your body? Is there anything you would you add?*

- gazing down or averting eyes
- covering face or body
- bowing head
- shrinking down
- collapse of body
- turning inward for long periods
- numbness
- compressing body
- extreme intensity
- difficulty breathing
- feeling hot or flushed
- quick flash/slow burn
- softer, dampened speech
- pain in pit of stomach

Continue to reflect on your memory and drawing of shame and compare your experience with this list of common impacts and effects of shame. If you are in a small group, share with another person.

Common effects and after-effects of shame
- wanting to disappear
- sense of dread

- appeasing or over-apologizing
- rage or depression
- hopelessness
- avoidance
- isolation
- feeling mortified
- distracting or impulsive behaviors
- inability to reality check
- loss of self-esteem and/or self-respect
- loss of sense of Self
- secrecy, denial, forgetfulness
- obsessiveness about what happened
- spiritual bereftness
- wish to die or disappear
- inability to accurately and objectively self-evaluate
- loss of access to emotional support
- dissociation and disorientation
- alienation
- attacking or blaming others
- disgust or contempt
- feeling of banishment or abandonment
- loss of internal resources for relating and self-care
- self-preoccupation
- loss of confidence
- self-loathing and self-attack
- outward rage or attack

Right Use of Power Teacher, Magi Cooper, graphically describes the experience of being in shame as akin to being a shore bird stuck in an oil slick. The oil slick is not the bird's fault. The oil sticks, doesn't wash off and prevents the bird from flying.

The Four Most Potent Effects
1. Isolation
2. Loss of internal resources
3. Hopelessness
4. Inability to reality check
5. Self-hatred (implosion) or outer rage (explosion)

Kinds of Shame

The feeling of unredeemable disgrace has many dimensions to be aware of. Some, as named by Robert Karen,[lxix] are:

- body shame
- situational shame
- competence shame
- relationship shame
- [cultural shame]
- [racial shame]
- [religious shame]

In all forms of shame people flash back to the core shame experience of irreparable disgrace, badness, or unlovableness. The immediate loss of connection, resources, and self-esteem make shame a very dramatic and disempowering emotion.

Responses to shame[lxx]

Our individual shame responses are scripts that have evolved over time to meet uncomfortable feelings, says Nathanson[lxxi] in his book, *Shame and Pride*. He identifies four types of response on two axis: time, and space. The time axis has its extremes—Withdrawal (a quick, sudden disconnection) and Avoidance (slow, distracting behavior which takes one away from the situation). The spatial axis redefines relationships and is between Attack Self (control the discomfort by taking control of the resultant bad feelings) and Attack Other (make someone else responsible). This range of responses explains the variety of strategies used by caregivers when they are operating from shame.

Shame and Trauma: The potency of shame makes it a traumatic experience. As with extreme fear or anxiety, shame disengages people from the social engagement nervous system[lxxii] that provides them with the interpersonal and internal connections and resources needed to deal with a situation without reverting to fight, flight, or freeze responses.

Guilt and Remorse: Guilt is a strong feeling of regret and sorrow for your own behavior that you feel and know caused harm. When experiencing guilt, people may be able to stop what they are doing. They can respond to feedback and organize around altering their behavior. Guilt can be moved toward the healing experience of regret. When feeling regret, people are resourced. They can acknowledge and take responsibility for causing harm, feel sorrow, and seek ways to self-correct. Regret or remorse heals and re-connects. A student[lxxiii] says, *"I think guilt is a feeling that assists us in finding our edge, or what is not quite right. It* *is a barometer for learning. If the lesson is missed, guilt can either turn inward: shame, or turn outward: blame. The point is to get the lesson before it has to introject or project."* Guilt is about behavior, while shame is about identity. Guilt returns a person to his or her own moral values and repositions his or her moral compass. When in the shame dungeon, however, consciousness, empathy and moral values are hidden, denied, or rejected. Right Use of Power teacher, Magi Cooper summarizes the difference between shame and guilt in this way:

SHAME	GUILT
unhealthy	healthy
immobilize	move forward
I am a mistake	I made a mistake
irredeemable	redeemable
personhood	behavior

Sorrow and Anger: For those who have been shamed and/or hurt, part of the healing process includes feeling sorrow and redirecting responsibility for the wound from Self to the abuser through appropriately expressed anger. This anger can be expressed non-violently and for the purpose of healing release with a therapist, colleague, or friend.

Self-Righteousness: Self-righteousness is the cousin of shame. Self-righteousness overrides compassion and makes it difficult to own our potential for causing harm. Genuine expressions of guilt, sorrow, and regret may deepen into shame if met with self-righteousness.

History

Shame, in the middle ages in Europe, was the primary force used to tame and control behavior. According to the research of Johan Huizinga.[lxxiv] *"The average European town dweller was wildly erratic and inconsistent, murderously violent when enraged, easily plunged into guilt, tears and pleas for forgiveness, and bursting with physical and psychological eccentricities.* Robert Karen[lxxv] adds, *"Situational shame spread rapidly, taming and civilizing the medieval passions, as a freer, more mobile society demanded that people be able to demonstrate to the world of strangers that they had their sexual and aggressive impulses on a leash."*

Now shame is no longer seen as the sole force around which inner controls are taught and organized. Caregivers are more motivated by empathy, altruism, spirituality, or social responsibility. These motivators are effective because they avoid the disconnect and loss of self-esteem that accompanies shame. Tragically, many law suits, prison systems, interrogation processes, parenting techniques, and educational methods still use shaming for behavior control and motivation for being good, despite demonstrations of shame's ineffectiveness for control and motivation.

There is on-going dialogue about whether the experience of shame over deeply inappropriate or harmful behavior has intrinsic benefit or no benefit at all. Indeed shame is an effective form of gaining immediate control. In this way it is similar to violence. But the harm this method of control causes is deep and costly as described in this chapter. I don't believe that the benefit of immediate control is worth the long-term costs.[lxxvi]   Further, because of the extreme effects of shame-- disconnection, sense of irreparable disgrace, self-loathing, and inability to reality check--there can be no such thing as "good" shame. Shame sufferers need to de-activate their shame before they can accurately assess their experience. Then, if their shame is a result of their own behavior, guilt can provide the guidance for self-correction and repair.

De-activating shame

You may have noticed that in the depths of the experience of shame, people are unable to determine whether they are abuser or abused, whether they have been hurt or caused hurt. For example, men or women who have been in a sexual relationship with a person in a position of trust often believe that it is their fault in some way. The universal experience of shame is that we are irreparably bad and disgraced. When we feel irreparably disgraced, we can't imagine the possibility of healing, and therefore, there is no reason to be accountable. Shame that is prolonged produces rage, deep depression or both.

Here's a chart to help you in sorting out what is needed to de-activate the impacts of shame. By using this chart, you may assist your clients (or Self or colleagues) to move from the universal shame experience to the universal experience of reconnection, first by recognizing and de-activating shame and then working through either of the pathways.

The pathway depends upon whether your client is the abuser or the abused. Notice that connecting with a compassionate listener and reality assessing are common to both routes. Shame and shaming are not healing and compassionate emotions. They fester in the unconscious. Neither healing nor remorse is accessible until shame is de-activated. Other feelings, such as grief, connectedness, and sorrow, are available when shame has been de-activated. These are useful for healing and self-correction.

> **Re-connection
> with Self, others, and reality**

• To let go, heal, and move on

• Openness to receive reparation and/or apology, and to be forgiving

• Regained ability to be connected

• Restored self-respect and empowerment

• Opportunity to grieve and heal

• Safe place to express anger, blame, resentment, betrayal

**to de-activate shame
of the one harmed**

• To heal, grow, and move on

• Openness to self-correct and offer reparation, and to be forgiven

• Regained ability to be connected

• Restored self-respect and self-worth

• Opportunity to successfully deal with underlying issues.

• Safe place to express remorse, guilt, regret, sorrow

**to de-activate shame
of the one causing harm**

then do a Reality check

• Connection with a compassionate, non-judgmental listener and then....

•Simple body movements—
arms and legs, large muscle group release,
activating all senses—
breathing in, moving head to re-orient—
humming, speaking, touch, eye contact—
imagining following a string of lights going up a set of stairs—

time moving forward
what's needed to get up out of the shame dungeon

> **Shame Dungeon**

Further detail about working with shame

- Getting out of shame and treating it takes a certain amount of bravery. First, learn to recognize shame in yourself and in your clients. Shame secretly rules many people's lives. Seek to normalize shame.

- The basics for de-activating shame come from deliberately moving the person from freeze mode to run or hit mode to the social engagement nervous system. This involves simple activities such as moving arms and legs, and activating senses by humming or speaking, touch, and making eye contact.

- Learn to deal with shame in the moment. When feeling shamed, notice your tendency to look down or away. Looking away is one of the indicators of the presence of shame.

- Next, acknowledge the shame. Speak it aloud, write it down or tell a trusted friend/ therapist/ mentor. Compassionate acknowledgement begins the process of recovery and may take the wind out of rage or depression.

- Remind yourself that when in the shame experience, you or your client is automatically unable to connect, resource, and reality check. Don't shame yourself for feeling de-resourced.

- Understand that, although you or your client has misused power or been abused by power, you or they are not irredeemably disgraced, or irreparably evil, flawed, or unlovable. The power of shame is in the association with your identity. When you can separate shame from identity, it becomes workable and steps can always be taken toward repair.[lxxvii]

- Get support. Don't isolate even though you feel shut down. Connect with someone and stay connected.

- Unburden by telling the story. Get the secret(s) out where it can be checked with reality. Sometimes people get "stuck" in repeating the story over and over again. They need some help in letting go.

- Learn how to make amends.

- Learn to revise internal dialogue from negative and shaming to positive and nurturing.

- Engage in the process of finding compassion, coming back into relationship, reawakening resources, and restoring self-worth.

- Once reconnected and resourced, you or your client can engage in accurate reality checking, healing, and restoring confidence, self-respect, and self-worth.

- Explore the possibility and healing power of forgiveness when the level of healing is appropriate. (See page 198 for guidance.)

Self-study Practice: Shame and the power spiral

1. De-Activating Shame

Ask a partner to do this process with you or proceed as a self-reflection. First, do the self-study process described on page 118. Or begin by looking again at the drawing, or notes, you previously made and remembering the shame event. Now, either with a partner or on your own, turn to each of the directions on the power spiral map. The following description is meant to serve as a guide for your process of practicing coming out of shame. When you are the bridge person assisting and receiving your partner (or yourself) back from their experience of shame, find a place of compassion and warmth and be present with your partner or yourself.

In the East, you recognize through both physiological and emotional features, that you are experiencing shame. Remind yourself that your felt sense is a common and universal response.

In the South, bring awareness to your experience; remembering and acknowledging that in the shame dungeon you are incapable of connecting, being resourced, feeling hopeful, or reality checking innocence or fault.

Now, turning to the West, imagine facing a partner with your eyes closed or your gaze downward. Take your time and do whatever you need to prepare yourself for reconnection and returning to reality. You may need to do simple things like moving your arms and/or legs a bit, or activating your senses by humming. Let your eyes be your bridge across. When you're ready, open your eyes briefly until you can keep them open and connected with your partner. You may have to open and close your eyes a number of times on your journey back. Next be open to anything else that may want to happen between you—a hand or hug, an unburdening of the story, hearing some important words.

Find a way to move to the North aspect with your partner or in your mind, gather insight and wisdom from your experience and let go of whatever is ready to be released. You may also want to draw this.

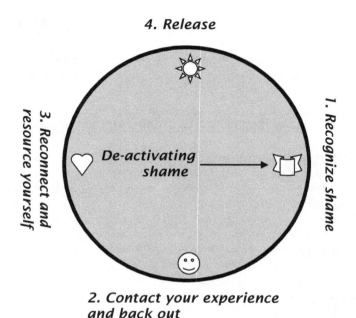

4. Release

**2. Contact your experience
and back out**

Having understood the dynamics of shame and learned to recognize it
and de-activate it, you and your clients will find many benefits.

- Heartfelt and compassionate regret
- Accurate self-evaluation and ability to reality check
- Empowerment to take appropriate responsibility
- Ability to better tolerate shame, shaming, and personal mistakes or
failings
- Ability to recognize shame and shaming and choose to maintain
eye contact, remain empowered, or leave the situation without loss
of self
- Less secrecy, rage, and/or depression
- Possibility of asking for or offering forgiveness

These are some responses to the experience of practicing de-activating shame:

- "I found just saying the word "shame" very freeing. It is good to name it what it is. It's as if I've created my own story from past shame that I bring into the present that has nothing to do with present experience."

- "When in the shame experience, my breath was short and it was literally impossible to smile."

- "I found myself feeling my feet on the earth and growing myself big. I needed my breath to fill myself up."

- "Coming out of shame was an act of will. It took wings of faith."

- "This is how I feel all the time! But I never had a name for it. What a relief."

2. Sources of Shame

Take a few moments to reflect on where your experiences of shame have come from. Here are some possibilities:

> school
>
> parents
>
> advertising
>
> legal system
>
> religion
>
> educational system
>
> corporate culture
>
> military

Non-Ordinary States

A non-ordinary state of consciousness is a "mild to deep trance in which awareness is focused in a different way than in ordinary life."[lxxviii] A student says:

"I'm amazed! It never occurred to me that my clients are often in a non-ordinary, mindful state of consciousness that needs even more sensitivity than usual. Thanks for pointing this out. This will translate immediately into more skillfulness and likely more effectiveness with my clients."

We all have experiences of non-ordinary states of consciousness, some very pleasurable and some traumatic. Non-ordinary states of consciousness engender special concerns about the right use of power because the impact of the power differential is heightened and expanded when clients are in a non-ordinary state. Thus, greater sensitivity and skillfulness in understanding and using your increased role power and influence for promoting well-being is needed.

Non-ordinary states can arise through experiences that are:

Pleasurable
> peak experience
> lovemaking
> religious experience
> sports, art, music, dance

Unpleasant
> shame
> pain
> grief
> traumatic experience or memory
> hypoglycemia
> sleep deprivation

Both or either
> mindfulness or present felt experience
> meditation
> emotional release

dissociation
fasting
drugs

As caregivers, we work with clients on a continuum of states of consciousness. This continuum moves from ordinary everyday states; to mild reverie[lxxix] in which our clients are relaxed, thoughtful, focused internally, and able to respond to questions; to deep, non-ordinary states as described in the self-study section. Clients may move fluidly along this continuum or make sudden shifts requiring attentive tracking.

Self-Study: Shifting your focus

Shift your focus to your present felt experience, get comfortable, close your eyes, and take a few breaths. Now recall a not too overwhelming memory of a time when you were in a non-ordinary state. Notice your experience. Use the following questions to help you access more deeply.
   "How do you experience your boundaries-where are they, how strong do they feel," etc.?
   "What's the focus of your attention?"
   "What is your level of vulnerability?"
   "How much awareness of your body do you have?"
   "What level of sensitivity to the environment, sound, and your intuitive abilities are you experiencing?"

Here's a list of some of the qualities and effects of non-ordinary experience.[lxxx] Which ones do you recognize?

- time distortion
- increased intensity of feeling and sensation
- greater need or capacity for faith and trust
- increased sensitivity and awareness through all senses
- consciousness expansion
- relaxation or diffusion of boundaries
- increased felt sense of the "truth"
- increased sensitivity to authenticity

One person's description of a non-ordinary state: "I had an extreme non-ordinary state experience during an attack by a man who tried to rape and kill me. I entered a transcendent state where I experienced little pain although I had recently had major abdominal surgery and I was trying to fight someone off of me who weighed about 300 pounds and was well over 6 feet tall. I was very calm and focused on the transcendent nature of the event and felt very protected and guided by a spiritual force. I could feel his emotional state with great awareness and my focus was on his emotional pain. I was near death for a while as he suffocated me and I had a very heightened state of consciousness as I felt myself leaving my body while receiving clear information about my lifetime."

Some of the most effective, profound, and long-lasting change and healing happens in a non-ordinary state. A colleague of mine, Anna Cox[lxxxi], says, "*I truly believe that deep healing happens primarily in non-ordinary states and that a therapist must be able to enter and relate comfortably to clients in these states with facility. Sometimes the non-ordinary state is the depth of the connection, and sometimes it is meditative, and sometimes it comes from intensity of feeling.*"

Since psychotherapy, body therapy, and massage are designed for the most part, to help people focus their awareness in an altered, internal state, clients may be in non-ordinary states more often than we think.

Influences of Non-Ordinary States

In addition to the qualities already described, other changes occur that effect the helping relationship.

- potential for stronger and more complicated transference and counter-transference
- greater suggestibility
- greater need for safety
- increased possibility of triggering the therapist's own fears and longings
- greater need for helping the client back into ordinary consciousness
- greater need to integrate profound experiences, especially when the client experiences cognitive dissonance

By learning to understand and accommodate to these changes we are better able to protect the client's spirit. It is essential to know how a non-ordinary state is being experienced by your client, and how non-ordinary states fit into the conceptual framework of your form of healing work in order to make effective interventions, adjustments, and assessments.

A psychotherapist, Susan Mikesic,[lxxxii] describes some feedback she received from a client: *"Ruth is very liable to enter an altered state during our meetings. Ruth game me some feedback once that was very helpful. She asked me not to talk at certain points during our sessions when she was deep inside herself. She described to me a dance performance she saw once where the dancers were dressed in colors that blended with the background so completely that they would disappear into the background whenever they stood still. It was only when they moved that you could even see them. Ruth told me that when I speak during certain moments of our sessions, I become like the moving dancer and she pays attention to me rather than to what she is seeing inside herself. [I now understand that a] person in an altered state is very much like the Princess in the fairy tale about the Princess and the Pea."*

Adjustment Suggestions

Here are some suggestions for making appropriate and effective adjustments when your clients are experiencing non-ordinary states. [lxxxiii]

- Pay especially close attention to setting boundaries for privacy, time, non-interference of outside sounds, energy, interruptions, and for safety and security needs.

- Keep in mind greater client suggestibility. Use direct, simple, clear language.

- Be spacious, slow down your pace, take plenty of time, allow for silence.

- Be especially cautious about giving advice. Clients in non-ordinary states are particularly open to and impacted by suggestions.

- Keep in mind that a regressed client has a need for simplicity and just being in their present felt experience of sensations and feelings. Don't use complicated or theoretical language.

- Be sensitive about the therapeutic use of touch. The experience of touch in a non-ordinary state tends to be more profound—often more needed, and often more easily confused with inappropriate touch.

- Allow time for the delicate transition back to ordinary consciousness. While in a non-ordinary state, experience may be transformative and dramatically healing, but integrating this

experience and new awareness into ordinary life may be
challenging and require time.

- Be self-aware. "A therapist's fear, lack of personal knowledge, and
  insufficient faith in the process may communicate itself to their
  client preventing their client from going fully into the experience
  to complete it."[lxxxiv]
- Learn how to distinguish between a healing process in a non-
  ordinary state and a process in which your client is being re-
  traumatized.
- Be alert to not intruding, over-intervening, over-reacting, over-
  interpreting, or pushing.
- Track and attend to your own fears or concerns, and arrange for
  supervision as needed. You may find that there are client
  experiences, perceptions, and beliefs that are difficult for you to
  affirm or attend to such as; past-life experiences, ritual abuse,
  multiplicity, ecstatic states, out of body experiences, near-death
  experiences, spiritual visions, kindling experiences, reliving birth,
  images of UFO abduction, or existential contemplation of suicide.

A colleague describes how she works with her clients in this
realm. "I often gently ease clients into non-ordinary states with
reassurance along the way and allow them to go as deeply or as
slowly as they are comfortable. I reassure them that I won't push
them, and that they can go into that state as they are ready. I don't
give them much intellectual information before or after and just
treat such states as part of their normal experience and nothing
unusual."[lxxxv]

In non-ordinary states, heightened and expanded sensory, emotional,
and spiritual experiences provide a context for very profound healing and
self-discovery, and also require special sensitivity to the increased impact
of the power differential.

Therapeutic Use of Touch

Story: Nancy's client Elena had seemed quite comfortable with touch.
She always asked for a hug at the end of the session and was readily able
to access body information. During one session she got in touch with a
deep longing for connection and began weeping. Nancy gently reached her
hand out and put it on Elena's knee to offer comfort. Elena quickly said in
a sharp tone, "Don't touch me!" Nancy was surprised and quickly
apologized and removed her hand, thanking Elena for telling her she
didn't want to be touched. Elena responded that she knew that it was okay
to say what she needed. Nancy then offered a self-study experiment of
offering her hand and inviting Elena to move her hand toward Nancy's
stopping when she began to get anxious. Nancy noticed that Elena was
rubbing the fingers of her other hand with her thumb as she moved her
right hand closer to Nancy's outstretched hand. Elena said that her left
hand was acting as both a guard against harm and a guide reminding her
what good touch feels like. Elena slowly moved her right hand, stopping
several times to check for safety, until she lightly touched the tips of
Nancy's fingers for a minute or so. As Nancy watched, Elena began
weeping, moved her fingers gently away, looked at Nancy and said, "I
stayed....and it was okay."

Touch is necessary to both physical health and emotional well-being.
Babies who aren't touched enough, fail to thrive. My colleague, Greg
Johanson[lxxxvi] is willing to go so far as to say that not to use the power of
touch (therapeutically and appropriately initiated) is itself unethical.
Restoring a satisfying and healthy relationship to touch may be indeed
considered a worthy goal in therapy. The body is a rich source of wisdom.
The use of body information and informed and conscious touch are
powerful tools for healing, self-awareness, establishing good boundaries,
and cultivating more satisfying connections.

Years of cultural, theoretical, and ethical controversy surround the use
of touch in the helping professions. In many states using touch is illegal
and/or uninsurable. The United States Association for Body Psychotherapy
(USABP) is an organization focusing on the therapeutic value of including
the body and ethical touch in healing work. A purpose of the USABP is to

increase the attention, validation and respect afforded to the modalities of body psychotherapy.

Ethical Codes for Helping Professions and State Laws related to the use of touch vary greatly. Please take responsibility for researching those Codes and Laws that are relevant in your place of residence.

Controversy arises from the following factors:

1) It is never ethical to use sexual touch with a client or to engage in or imply sexual intimacy or the future possibility of such.[lxxxvii] The very strong healing power of touch is matched by the equally strong harm caused by sexual intimacy in a relationship of trust. The prohibition of even non-sexual touch in helping relationships by organizations is intended to prevent the egregious harm caused by inappropriate touch.

2) Human beings automatically and uniquely assign meaning to touch. Thus, therapeutic touch is easily misinterpreted by clients as sexual, forceful, caregiver-serving or controlling. Touch is deeply longed for and a source of deep vulnerability. Use of therapeutic touch is ethically and relationally complex and requires assessment, sensitivity, good tracking, and clarity of intention on the part of caregivers.

The following information, much of it by Jaffy Phillips, MA[lxxxviii], is offered in support of the healing power of the therapeutic use of touch. It can be a guide to how to assess the appropriateness of touch, set up the use of touch, and track for the impact of the use of touch. Ms. Phillips has set these guidelines for the use of touch in psychotherapy, but the information, considerations, and applications are helpful for caregivers in general.

Value of the therapeutic use of touch[lxxxix]

The therapeutic use of touch may be considered when a caregiver assesses any of the following to be client needs:

- To establish a sense of connection or contact with the therapist.
- To communicate acceptance and "touchability" (thus relieving shame and isolation).
- To explore and strengthen the client's boundaries.
- To explore the client's history in relation to touch and/or intimacy.
- To promote the client's awareness of his or her body.
- To promote cognitive and emotional insight through direct felt experience of issues.
- To support or contain the expression of emotion.

- To calm and retrain the client's nervous system in the context of trauma history.
- To help the client complete truncated developmental processes.
- To help a client ground and come into greater contact with reality.
- To focus or direct a client's attention.
- As a natural expression of the therapist's caring.
- There are some clients for whom touch is a central issue, and for whom restoring a satisfying relationship to touch may be a central focus of the therapy. These include clients who have been physically or sexually abused and clients with intimacy and closeness issues.
- Touch is often used to help provide a corrective emotional experience in reparation of early abusive or neglectful environments.
- Touch brings consciousness to the body.
- Touch brings the therapist and client into present moment experience.
- Touch is an effective communication for kinesthetic learners.
- Touch encourages the client to honor the wisdom of their body and demonstrates a practical way to access that wisdom.
- Touch helps the client develop internal somatic tracking skills.
- Touch quiets physical and mind noise that often over-rides awareness.
- Touch feels good.

Touch supports the process of therapy as it...

- Enhances feelings of closeness and trust with the therapist.
- Enhances self-disclosure.
- Increases risk-taking and self-exploration.
- Engages clients more fully in the therapeutic process.
- Helps clients to tolerate pain and shame while working through deep issues.
- Enhances client's self-esteem.

- Offers another sense besides hearing and seeing to reinforce therapeutic messages
- Helps bring client into present felt experience

Assessing for the use of touch

"When you touch someone, everything changes." Touch is a physical and relational experience that is generally imbued with layers of historical, cultural, and psychological meaning. The meanings evoked by touch are often unconscious or non-verbal, and they often manifest somatically and/or relationally before the client is able to articulate anything about them. Boundary violation, transference, and counter-transference are the most common examples of this kind of response; unaddressed, these issues can wreak havoc in the therapeutic relationship and ultimately damage the client. When considering the use of touch, the following categories are important considerations.

Boundaries and intimacy

Touching is an intimate act and one that carries the potential to invade the client's boundaries and/or to trigger strong transferential reactions. It can also be a confusing and/or overwhelming experience for a client with poor boundaries or a poorly developed sense of self.

Client individuality

There are only very general guidelines about the kinds of client populations for whom touch is indicated or contraindicated. Within these categories, each client is individual, and each therapist/client dyad has its own unique characteristics in terms of the quality of the relationship as well as the transferences and counter-transferences present.

Variability of meaning

The same kind of touch will be experienced by different clients in different ways, depending on the circumstances, the client's personal history and cultural background, personal qualities of the therapist, and the quality and duration of the therapeutic relationship. It is important that the therapist avoid re-enacting negative aspects of the client's interpersonal or touch history and/or reinforcing any of the client's negative associations to touch.

Protection of the client

It is only ethical to use touch with a client when it is both clinically advisable and used in the context of informed consent. With many clients, asking permission to touch is not enough. Because of the impact of the power differential, clients may want to be good or compliant, and may say "yes" when meaning "no," or may not disclose when the touch feels uncomfortable, confusing, or triggering. Practitioners who use touch need to be very attentive to non-verbal as well as verbal signals from the client.

Self-protection

The potential for misunderstanding of the use of touch in psychotherapy is high. Our cultural norms, in combination with Freud's legacy (the touch taboo in psychotherapy) support the interpretation of all touch as sexual and/or invasive. Given the complexity of the therapeutic relationship, the power differentials that exist, and the unknowns of the client's history, it is wise to proceed with caution.

History of abuse

Clients for whom touch is a central issue include those who have been sexually or physically abused, or those who have a history of intimacy issues. In working with these clients, practitioners should proceed with extra care, tracking, and discretion in order to avoid reinforcing the client's negative associations with touch.

Dynamics and dimensions of touch[xc] for both therapists and body workers include:

- type
- quality
- location
- timing
- pressure
- how contact is made and exited
- how long the touch lasts
- whether there is movement after contact has been made
- whether verbal exchange accompanies touch

Guidelines for the Use of Touch

- Be well-informed about the guidelines for the use of touch that governs your modality and your region of practice.
- Add a "touch education" component to your intake interview.
- Obtain informed consent, both written and verbal. Discuss and document the following things:
  - Client knows how and why touch will be used in the therapy.
  - Client understands limits and boundaries of touch (e.g. non-sexual).
  - Client agrees to this and gives permission.

- Client knows that they can stop or discontinue the use of touch at any time, and that they are always in control of when, where, how, and for how long they are touched..
- Touch should always and only be used deliberately, carefully, and consciously.
- The use of touch should be accompanied by assessment and a clear clinical rationale.
- Take the time to become clear about your intentions and feelings towards your client. Lack of clarity about intentions is often a sign that shadow material or counter-transference is present.
- Become familiar with your own touch issues and potential counter-transferences.
- The use of touch should be accompanied by verbal processing of the client's experience.
- Be mindful: stop touching when your intention is complete.
- Stay within the limits of your competency (some kinds of touch require special training).

Avoid touch when...
- The therapist does not want to touch.
- The client does not want to be touched.
- The client is likely to misinterpret the touch.
- Either client or therapist feels that touch would not be helpful.
- The client is in a regressed state, if touch has not already been explicitly explored and contracted for as a way to provide grounding and reality contact.

To summarize the guidelines:
Therapeutic touch should be...

non-sexual	*mindful*
appropriate	*with permission*
conscious	*cautious*
well-boundaried	*uncontaminated by caregiver's personal needs*
in service of the client	*carefully tracked and contacted*
adjusted as needed	

Practitioners who want to begin using touch, might choose to use it first with couples, groups or families. Because there are others in the room, and the therapist is directing, not participating, touch is less likely to evoke transference issues or be misinterpreted.[xci]

General Assessment Factors for the Use of Touch

There are three aspects to consider and assess: client factors, caregiver factors, and relationship factors.

Client Factors
- History and issues, including touch history.
- Ego strength, level of functioning, diagnostic category.
- Relational dynamics.
- Cultural factors.
- Boundary awareness and ability to say "no," in general and to the therapist.
- Whether the client wants to be touched.
- Quality of eye contact.
- Quality of verbal contact.
- Quality of reality contact.
- Congruence of verbal and somatic presentation.
- Whether the use of touch is in accord with current client needs.

Therapist Factors
- Degree of appropriate training in using touch in a therapeutic context.
- Ability to maintain clear therapeutic intent and clear boundaries.
- Familiarity with the use of touch through own experiences in therapy.
- Knowledge and awareness of own relationship to touching and being touched, including potential counter-transference reactions.
- Attitude and feelings towards client.
- Degree of comfort with touch and physical closeness.
- Ability to manage client's potential sexual and/or emotional responses to the touch.
- Ability to access and make use of support including personal therapy, supervision, and peer support to process feelings and counter-transferences related to the use of touch.

- Whether the use of touch is congruent with the therapist's beliefs, attitudes, and values in the context of the present relationship

Therapeutic Relationship Factors
- Are the strength, length, and quality of the therapeutic alliance adequate?
- Has trust been established?
- Are the boundaries of the relationship understood?
- Is there sufficient openness in the relationship to process the client's responses to touch, which might include negative or ambivalent feelings towards the therapist?
- Would the physical intimacy of the touch exceed the level of emotional intimacy present in the relationship?
- Does either therapist or client experience the suggestion of touch as a demand?
- Is the client in control of all aspects of the physical contact?

Research Results: Client Evaluations[xcii]

I find the research reported here to be very revealing and useful because it comes directly from clients' self-reported and real-life experience.

Clients reported positive experiences of touch in therapy when...
1) There is clarity regarding the boundaries of therapy.
2) The touch is congruent with the level of intimacy in the relationship.
3) The client feels they are in control of the physical contact.
4) The client perceives that the touch is for his or her own benefit rather than the therapist's.
5) The particular use of touch is congruent with the client's issues.
6) The client perceives that the therapist is sensitive to the client's reaction to touch.
7) The client is able to communicate with the therapist about feelings towards the therapist.

Clients reported negative experiences of touch in therapy when. . . .
1) They felt trapped in the gratification of being close.
2) They felt guilty towards the therapist, whom they perceived as nurturing.
3) There was a reversal of roles, and they felt responsible for the therapist's well-being.

4) The relationship with the therapist was a recapitulation of the client's childhood family dynamics.

Potential for risk of sexual interpretation

Touch may be interpreted by a client as sexual contact. Minimize this risk by the following:

1) The presence of a clear contract about the use of touch.
2) Clarity about one's own intentions and motivations for touching a particular client at a particular time.
3) Clarity about one's own sexual boundaries.
4) Scrupulous use of supervision.
5) The client has tracking and reporting ability.
6) The ability of client and therapist to stay in truth.
7) The presence of client's partner, a co-therapist, or group members in the office.

Risk that touch will be used to gratify the needs of the therapist

Touch can be used to gratify other (non-sexual) needs, including the therapist's need for intimacy and closeness, need to be experienced as a nurturer by the client, and/or need for physical contact. Therapists can minimize the risk of this type of exploitation by becoming familiar with their own needs through personal therapy and self-awareness practices, establishing outside sources for their gratification, and regular use of supervision.

Signs of danger for helping professional

- Different quality or use of touch with different gendered clients.
- Touch used in an unexamined way in response to a client's request.
- Touch that occurs in secret, or with reluctance of the therapist to discuss their use of touch with colleagues or a supervisor.
- Touch that occurs in the context of sexual attraction, by either therapist or client.

An excellent reference for further study on this topic is: *The Ethics of Touch*, by Ben Benjamin and Cherie Sohnen-Moe.

The use of touch has a long history in the helping professions and serves as a cornerstone for many of the forms of work that are practiced today. **Wise and informed use of touch is well worth attention,**

validation, and support, and has great healing potential. It is a powerful intervention.

Developing somatic tracking skills will allow both you and your clients to monitor the impact of touch. With this information you will be able to explore your client's experience of touch in ways that can be meaningful and empowering to your clients. These several activities can help identify and heal aspects of your clients' relationship with touch and the interpersonal complexities that can arise as a result of the use of touch.

1. Awareness of the effect of touch

This activity (designed by Jim Kepner[xciii]) can be done by yourself or with a partner to highlight what touch brings to your experience.

First, rub your hands together and take a breath, letting it out. Take a moment now to notice your dominant hand and let yourself shift gently from wherever you are centered in your body to be fully present in your hand. Take a moment, too, to notice how you feel in your opposite forearm—the sensations and sense of presence, warmth and liveliness. Now, just gently, but with good contact, rest your palm on the opposite forearm. Take a moment to feel with your touching hand how you make contact, as you continue to breathe and feel. You might feel only the surface, cloth or skin. You might feel your arm as an object. You might feel your warmth, perhaps to begin to sense into your flesh and bone, blood and energy. This might be a simple meeting, or a profound remembrance.

Now shift your attention to your sense of being touched. What kind of touch does this part of you call for? Warmth, understanding, appreciation, firmness, stillness, movement? If you wish, you may shift how you are touching to match what the touched side of you is calling for and see what this is like.

2. Qualities and Intentions in Touch

This self-study[xciv] will help you increase your awareness and sensitivity to how different qualities and intentions are experienced physically and emotionally.

Either working with your own hand or with a partner, choose a shoulder, knee, or hand as the place to experience several qualities of touch. One at a time, each partner will mindfully touch the other with particular energetic qualities or intentions in mind. *These could be written on cards ahead of time so that the touch receiver doesn't know what the particular quality is.* Use some or all of the following: needy, clear, merged, distant/cold, sexual, fearful, and cautious. Receivers: study how you experience the differences and try to name the quality being transmitted. Touchers: study the responses of your receiver to each quality, both subtle and obvious responses. *Know in advance that you may be choosing to experience, for your learning, several uncomfortable qualities.*

3. Effects of Inappropriate Touch

This part of the exercise requires a partner. As receiver: *"Silently remember a time when you were touched either appropriately or inappropriately, and notice what the memory of that experience feels like emotionally and in your body. Please ask your unconscious to be a friend and offer you an incident with only a medium degree of charge, and one that is non-sexual."* As a giver: *"Sit with your partner and see what you notice happening in their body as they are remembering. Also track your own experience."* Now reverse roles and do the same process. Talk about your experience. What did you notice? What kinds of things did you track? How did you check it out? What kinds of assessment clues did you discover?

The intention here is to give you an opportunity to practice tracking and naming what you notice and to observe how much information is available without words.

Sexuality

Rev. John was the youth minister of a community church. One of the teenagers in his youth group came to him in great distress and tears of grief over the death of her beloved dog. Rev. John reached his hand out and put it on her shoulder to comfort her. She experienced this as a sexual advance and reported the incident to the church board. Was John unconsciously or consciously being sexual? Did John have unmet needs for intimacy in his life? Had the teenager been sexually wounded and thus triggered by any touch from a man? Was John not tracking her caution around touch and the impact of the touch so that he could resolve the situation before it escalated? Should John have asked her permission to comfort her with a gentle touch on her shoulder? Was the teenager having some other difficulty with John that she couldn't talk about?

These are the kinds of complex issues that arise around sexuality and touch. No wonder inappropriate sexual intimacy is a frequent category for ethical grievances! Sexual intimacy causes much of the significant ethical harm to clients. Strong societal judgment, shame, self-righteousness, and desire for revenge surround accusations of sexual abuse of power.

Sexual energy or sexual current is a normal, healthy, pleasurable and nourishing experience. In itself, it is not bad or shameful. Sexual intimacy is an expression of the human longing for love, cherishing, and nurturing. It is a significant human need; a profound biological urge; and a major gateway to a transcendent state of consciousness. Romantic fantasies of being desired and fully alive are deep and compelling.

Though sexuality is a natural part of life, it is how sexuality is misused that is harmful. Overt and covert sexual abuse, sexual disorders, sexual confusion, pornography, low self-esteem, poor societal and familial boundaries, and shame all contribute to the rampant sexual wounding in our world. **Egregious cases of sexual abuse of power by professionals absolutely must be handled through grievance processes and legal actions.**

The subtleties of intention and impact in sexual dynamics, unfortunately elude many practitioners. From research by Gabbard we find that *"although a percentage of abusing therapists is unquestionably predatory by design, studies indicate that a larger percentage become swept up in powerful transference-counter-transference enactments in which all perspective is lost and grossly misguided action occurs. . . [Other research by Carr and Robinson] indicates that the majority of sexually abusive therapists believe, in general, that sexual involvement with a patient is destructive but that somehow theirs was a special case that was not harmful and possibly was even therapeutic to their patient.* "[xcv] There are complex reasons for such misguided confusion. A few are named here. Sexuality between people in helping relationships remains extremely   difficult to approach. We are called to compassion rather than shame.

Sexual feelings are experienced as difficult, vulnerable, embarrassing, shameful, and inappropriate as subjects of conversation. It is therefore very challenging for either caregiver or client to bring these feelings into the open. These feelings are also not often brought to supervision. When feelings like these are not talked about, they become exaggerated or repressed.

Clients may interpret a therapist's compassionate acceptance as sexual attraction. Clients who confuse sex with love, such as those with sexual abuse in their backgrounds are especially at risk. Therapists may also confuse the therapeutic closeness with a desire for sexual intimacy. As Kottler and Van Hoose put it, *"An ethical therapist realizes that clients are unusually susceptible to feelings of adoration for their therapists, and that affection can be translated into sexual desire."* [xcvi]

Caregivers may have unmet needs for intimacy that may unintentionally "leak" into their relationships with clients. Caregivers may have a poor, undeveloped, or inaccurate level of self-awareness about the impact of their behavior. They may not know when their behavior is experienced by clients as seductive. It is well to remember that most practitioners will in great likelihood encounter these situations. The knowledge of the subtle impacts of the power differential is paramount in maintaining impeccability while putting aside personal needs.

Sexuality is a highly personal and private experience that is seldom talked about openly enough to normalize it. Because it is personal and private, and because it is rare to ask for and receive feedback about it, widely varied interpretations of the same covert or overt sexual behaviors that could erode ethical boundaries are rarely discussed.

Sexual current, being an essential life force, will be present in relationships. Because it is such a compelling energy, it is challenging, but worth the effort to learn how to normalize so these sexual feelings can be understood and sublimated so that the practitioner doesn't take advantage of clients.

Sexual intimacy, an emotional affair, or language or behavior that is seductive, suggestive, demeaning, exploitative, or harassing is never appropriate in any relationship with a power differential.[xcvii] *"Regardless of any conceivable benefits from sexual encounters, it is incomprehensible that the possible side effects, problems and complications could ever justify this activity. Certainly, the therapist would lose the needed sense of objectivity and neutrality necessary to be helpful, not to mention the exploitive, oppressive and manipulative implications. Sex with clients only further confuses a relationship that is already unequal in power and control."*[xcviii]

Inappropriate and harmful sexual activity includes any physical or verbal behavior that is suggestive, seductive, harassing, demeaning, exploitative. And emotional affair is also harmful. The client's attraction to the therapist can be therapeutically discussed as long as (a) boundaries are held extremely clearly (including explicit agreement that there is no possibility of sexual relationship now or in the future), (b) therapist is not being excessively affected by attraction or counter-transference, (c) therapist focuses on client's sexual issues only to the extent that such discussion is based on the client's therapeutic process.

This is a highly sensitive issue that deserves open and honest self-reflection. Here are some things to consider when examining sexual feelings toward or from clients.

Coping with Sexual Feelings Toward a Client

1) Explore why you are attracted to this particular client. Is there something about this person that meets a need that should be met elsewhere?

2) Seek out an experienced colleague who can help you sort this out and take appropriate action.

3) Seek personal counseling, to help you resolve your feelings about this client and to uncover the issues in your life that you may not be dealing with.

4) If you are unable to resolve your feelings appropriately, terminate the professional relationship and refer the client to another therapist.

Coping with Sexual Feelings From a Client

1) Acknowledge your clients' feelings as normal. Appreciate their courage and vulnerability around bringing it up or having it named. Explain that the kind of intimacy that often develops in a client/therapist relationship is powerful and can easily be interpreted as sexual. The love experienced is actually a kind of contextual love that is specific to the power differential relationship. Sexualizing this kind of love is detrimental to the therapeutic relationship.

2) Make it explicitly clear, in both your words and your body language that a sexual relationship is outside the boundaries of the therapeutic relationship. (Ethical codes vary in their statements of when (if ever) after termination it is considered ethical to begin a sexual relationship.)

3) Make every effort not to shame or reject your client, and track for and attend to any signs of shame or rejection.

4) If appropriate, look for therapeutic ways in which the sexuality issue could be worked as a therapeutic issue.

5) When these feelings are unspoken or unconfirmed, you need to use your best professional judgment about whether it would be most in service of your client to name the feelings or to leave the choice up to your client.

6) Be prepared in advance. Consider how you would handle this kind of situation; or how you can handle it more skillfully. Seek the support of supervision.

Deepening Understanding

The issue of sexuality goes much deeper than simply understanding and setting boundaries. Here are several questions brought up by students that can help you deepen your understanding.

- *When a client tells me they are attracted to me, I feel flattered and awkward. How can I express myself so that the attention doesn't end up on me and my response, or so my client doesn't get the wrong impression?*

- *How do I work with clients who automatically associate intimacy with sexuality?*

- *Must I shut down my sexuality altogether to be an ethical therapist or body worker?*

- *How can I help a client understand the difference between therapeutic or transpersonal love and personal love?*
- *What are right and wrong uses of sexual current?*
- *Can sexual current itself be separated out from therapeutic love and intimacy? Or is it just to be "managed," understood and accepted?*
- *Should the experience of sexual current in a session always be named?*
- *How can I tell when a client is misunderstanding my intention?*
- *What is the range of control over my sexual feelings that I personally and realistically have?*
- *How can I effectively and appropriately use this control?*
- *Is there a way this client's attraction could be used therapeutically?*

Potential for therapeutic use of touch to lead to or be interpreted as sexual contact

The risk that touch will lead to sexual contact or will be misinterpreted can be minimized by:

- The presence of a clear contract such as described in the chapter on therapeutic use of touch.

- Clarity about your intentions and motivations for touching a particular client at a particular time.

- Clarity about the absolute boundaries of "no sexual contact with clients", and commitment to keeping these boundaries.

- A willingness to examine feedback about your unconscious effect on clients.

- Meticulous use of supervision.

A few stories:

• *"A male counselor was attracted to a female client. He knew she was in crisis. He offered to meet her in a restaurant to provide professional support. She was in a vulnerable position having just gone through a nasty divorce where her ex-husband had numerous affairs. She talked about feeling unlovable and unattractive. The counselor placed his arm around her shoulder to comfort her and offered to follow her home to check on her safety. After nurturing and supporting her, they slipped into a sexual situation."* This counselor has taken advantage of his client's vulnerability and has likely been led more by unmet personal needs and poor boundaries and poor judgment than malicious intent to harm. Sexuality is a strong motivator, and can warp normal ability to make good judgments, and as a friend says, "Please stay away. My hands grow larger and my head smaller when love is before me." [xcix]

• A caregiver writes: *"My point of view is that what we need most of in this world is love. This is what motivates my work and I believe it is the fundamental of all healing energies. When I sign a note to a client, "love," I am not worried about people personalizing it with me since everyone knows or senses that I am not being romantic or suggestive. I think we are all adults here. And I still call my clients, "darling" sometimes. No one gets the wrong idea."* Compelling, but, in fact, people everywhere, and especially people when in a Down-power role, <u>do</u> get the wrong idea, <u>do</u> misinterpret, <u>do</u> make words mean something they want them to mean, and <u>do</u> confuse personal and transpersonal love when they are vulnerable and longing for love and acceptance.

• As part of a process of relationship repair between a student and a teacher, the student explained her experience. *"I was confused by how you related to me in terms of your body language and energy when we met at a restaurant to talk about some theoretical questions I had. Your words and lack of help in focusing me and our conversation on the question created more and more confusion and insecurity within me. I felt ashamed of these feelings. Then when you sat down next to me at the table, instead of across from me, I felt invaded and manipulated. I felt uncomfortable and expressed my discomfort and vulnerability with the "newness" of being with a man, and in particular a single man in this type of context. It felt more like a date than a teacher-student meeting. I felt ignored and disregarded when you failed to respond to my concern and discomfort. I began to feel that your needs were more important, and I feel angry now as I see that I was subtly forced to push my needs aside in order to stay in relationship with you and get my question answered. I needed you to maintain the boundary between us a teacher and student because I couldn't do it myself. I trusted you, and this trust was violated. My shame prevented me from resourcing myself and correcting the situation, but I hold you responsible for seeing this and doing something about it in order to care for me and protect my spirit as a vulnerable student and single woman."* The courage and clarity of both the student and the teacher in facing this situation enabled clarity and resolution. The teacher understood, apologized, and did some therapeutic work in understanding his boundary issues and lack of sensitivity and responsiveness to his impact.

• A college teacher describes a powerful learning experience: *As a professor, I had a profound experience of temptation, confusion, and challenge. To my dismay, I found myself very attracted to one of the male students in a new class. I had been single for many years and was particularly vulnerable to sexual energy directed toward me. This student was very warm and delightful and actively engaged in the class. Exuding sexual innuendo, he would come up to me after class and compliment me. He asked me out to lunch, and knowing this was inappropriate, I said "no." But my feelings of attraction to him were growing. To my amazement, I actually found myself thinking, "He's really a good match for me. I have been looking for so long. I know it is unethical to get involved with a student, but for true love, it would be worth it, and I could just quit my job." I happily consulted with my department head, thinking that she would agree with me and support me in my plan. Nope. And thank goodness she did not agree! She was quite firm: "Don't you dare do this. You are an excellent teacher and it would be too big a loss for us and for you to quit teaching. And it would be very harmful to this student and to the rest of the class." It took a few moments, but sanity and my desire not to cause harm returned and I agreed not to go there.*

However, then I had to figure out what to do with this very strong sexual attraction. As I sat with it, I understood that attraction happens beyond my choice, but how I respond to attraction is within my power. So I set about consciously withdrawing my attraction. This was something I could use my will to do. Empowering. I thought that would be the end of the story. But the student came to me and said, "Have I done something wrong? You are so different with me. You are now cold and distant instead of warm." I was now causing another kind of harm. I'm glad that he was willing to risk talking with me directly. I decided to be authentic and told him that I was aware of feeling a strong sexual attraction to him and that I had needed to withdraw it because such a relationship was not appropriate with him as a student. I wanted him to understand and I trusted that I would be able, in time, to find a balanced place of response to him. He sat quietly for quite a while and then said, " I get it. But I want you to know that I don't feel a sexual attraction toward you. I feel a love for you as a teacher." How embarrassing, the whole thing was a projection! I sat for a while trying to compose myself. Big breath. "Well, that is good to know. Thank you for telling me. But that was a lot of energy you sent my direction. I misinterpreted. I'm curious about whether there is anything familiar here in your relationship to other teachers?" Silence. "Now that you are asking me to look at this, I see that it is a pattern I have. I try to charm teachers in order to make myself special. I guess I have something to withdraw too." There was something there for both of us. A normalized student and teacher relationship reorganized and emerged over time. This one worked out.

This teacher learned how easy it is to confuse personal and sexual love with the kind of love clients or students have for the up-power person. In the story, this kind of student love was admiration mixed with a habit of using charm. Reading her story makes it easier to understand how it happens that teachers so often get sexually involved with students or clients. These two kinds of love, personal and transpersonal, have a lot of similarities. The dynamic is further complicated by the desire of students to be special, and the additional influence that the power differential gives to the teacher. The teacher in this story also learned how important it is to talk over ethical dilemmas with colleagues or through supervision, especially when the issue is something about which you feel ashamed or is a mistake you have already made or might make. When personal sexual desires get involved, thinking can become very warped.

Self-Study

1. As you read the stories on the previous pages, what thoughts and feelings come up in you? Do you identify with any of the therapists? Do you identify with any of the clients? Would you have come to the same or different conclusions in either role?

2. The following exercise requires a partner. It involves some risk-taking, but gets experientially into the heart of exploring the complexities of sexual current.

Choose someone with whom you feel comfortable exploring this topic. Sit facing each other. You will be learning about the experiential differences of touch depending on your intention. Taking turns, simply holding your partner's hand, intend to convey your choice of any of the following attitudes and feelings. Tell your partner what you are intending to convey for the first two. Without telling your partner what you intended, try out two or more others on the list of intentions. Both partners mindfully study each experience and share what you each experience. Complete when you have enough information and talk together about your insights from the whole process. What can you take from this into your work with clients?

- feeling detached/objective
- feeling worried/concerned/fearful
- feeling compassionately accepting, loving presence
- feeling sexual attraction
- feeling needy for intimacy
- trying to stop or block sexual feelings
- feeling shame for having sexual feelings
- feeling universal, transpersonal love

Transference

Story: Greg, a new therapist, working toward licensure, had a strong need to be acknowledged as a good therapist. At the end of a session that was videotaped for supervision, as his client was quietly self-reflecting and beginning to re-orient, Greg said, "Well, I thought that was a really great session! Then, catching himself, he added, "But it's your session, you're the one who should decide." His client, having a strong need to be liked and a good client, reached out her hand to Greg's knee and said, reassuringly, "Yes, it was a great session." His supervisor could see (from a perspective not available to Greg who was not experiencing any difficulty in the relationship) that the unconscious transference and counter-transference was preventing the therapeutic relationship from deepening to the significant issues that needed attention. Greg was afraid of being unsuccessful, and his client was afraid of being rejected.

Transference

Transference is a normal phenomenon in relationships. With a power differential, transference is amplified. Transference in this context, refers to the process whereby clients project onto their therapist past feelings or attitudes they had toward significant people in their lives. Transference entails misperceptions of the professional, either positive or negative. These projections may lead to a repetition in the present of the ideas of relationships from past history. Transference patterns often can be used effectively as therapeutic issues.

Projection

Projection is a particular kind of transference. It involves repeating a real or fantasy relationship from the past. This is not a problem unless it is unconscious. As a caregiver, a signal that projection may be happening is that you feel you are being treated in a way that seems incongruent with what's happening. When projection is problematic, either you or your client is interacting as if the other was a person from the past. Projection has many degrees from harmless to serious disruption of ability to function in the world. When projecting, the person deals with emotional content that has external or internal stressors by falsely attributing to another his/her own unacceptable feelings. This can lead to acting on these ideas and a confused notion of what's real and what's not. Then you begin to believe the other is exactly like the person in your history. Projective identification is a self-fulfilling prophecy.

This chapter is not intended to be a replacement for an in-depth study of transference dynamics. Rather it is basic information that links transference to power and ethics. The potential positive or negative impact of transference is increased in power differential relationships. Transference issues often are subtle or unconscious and can thus create relationship confusion. Transferences and counter-transferences may also develop into dysfunctional client/caregiver systems.

Transference—both shadow and light—is one of the most important mechanisms at work in power dynamics. Transference and counter-transference are usually outside awareness. Thus, supervision is especially important and valuable in becoming conscious about these dynamics. The information in this chapter is focused toward psychotherapists, however, the transfererence patterns described here occur in other care-giving relationships.

The influence of the power differential increases client's vulnerability to several core human needs and longings that are very susceptible to both negative and positive transference. **These are the need and longing to be loveable and to love, and the need and longing to be worthy**. Belonging, feeling welcome, respected, and intrinsically valued are aspects of the above needs. The power differential also increases the vulnerability of caregivers in the same ways—from their need and longing to be liked and valued by their clients. Negative beliefs about personal "loveableness" and worth, fears of rejection and/or criticism, and unmet needs for feeling loved and worthwhile are common dynamics involved in both transference and counter-transference.

A second related dynamic associated with the power differential is the idealize/devaluing dynamic. Clients project an idealized image onto their caregiver. When the caregiver does something that is not ideal, he or she is devalued. This devaluing is typically stronger than the actual event warrants. Caregivers may find the idealizing surprising and the devaluing confusing. Clients may wish the therapist to be perfect.

Idealizing and de-valuing are complex dynamics. Often they are reflections of transference or the impact of the power differential. However, clients may be expressing genuine gratitude or authentic dissatisfaction that is the outcome of a healthy and empowered care-giving relationship. It is important to receive appreciation with warmth and self-nourishment. Giving appreciation is empowering for clients and for the relationship. Likewise, it is important to receive expressions of dissatisfaction with grace and openness. Responding well to dissatisfaction is also empowering for clients and the relationship. Sometimes it is challenging to discern appreciation and dissatisfaction from problematic transference. Sometimes it is challenging to respond skillfully to appreciation and dissatisfaction.

Normal aspect of relationships[c]

Transference and counter-transference often occur unconsciously, are universal, and occur to varying degrees in all relationships. Assume that it's happening. Both client and caregiver make unconscious interpretations and projections. Both client and caregiver have unconscious influence on each other. Being alert to these impacts helps caregivers be more sensitive to the effects of the power differential.

Neither the client nor caregiver can be fully aware of:

- *How they experience the other*
- *How the other is experiencing them*
- *How these experiences are influencing themselves or the other*

Universal Energy Field

Before discussing specific transference patterns, it is important to mention that one of the most potent ways to stay clear of problematic transference issues, is to be centered and aligned with the Universal Energy Field.[ci] Marcus Borg calls this field simply, "the more." "These non-religious terms could be used to describe the infinite energy we see in nature, the unlimited potentials that we enjoin in working with our clients, the consciousness that is greater than our personalities, or the vital life force that sustains us. The caregiver's alignment with the UEF, through centering permits her to disconnect from her ego needs or to see personal power as the source of healing. Instead, the healer establishes a sense of focused balance within her personal biofield. As the patient's more depleted field begins to respond to the focused intention of the practitioner, he may begin to connect to his energy source that permits him to experience his own gifts without over-dependency on the facilitator, and without unrealistic expectations."[cii] By centering and aligning with the UEF, or "the more" caregivers can often avoid the enmeshing of biofields that leads to problematic transference. Connecting with this encompassing "field" also resources and replenishes.

Transference Patterns[ciii]

These descriptions have focused on the problematic aspect of each of these transference patterns for the counselor. However, these dynamics also have an intrinsic value in helping relationships when not exaggerated. Watson describes some common transference patterns:

1) **Counselor as ideal.** The counselor is seen as a perfect person, without flaws, who does everything right. The client elevates the therapist, puts self down, and loses identity. The danger is that the counselor can come to believe these projections.

2) **Counselor as seer.** The counselor is seen as the expert, all knowing, all powerful. The client looks to the counselor for direction, answers. The danger is that the counselor can feed on the projection and subsequently give advice to the client that is based on the counselor's need to be the expert. There is also a danger that the counselor could encourage the client to remain dependent.

3) **Counselor as nurturer.** The client plays a helpless, small child and wants hugs and holding. The danger is that the counselor may become the nurturing parent and take care of the client, and the client will never learn personal responsibility.

4) **Counselor as frustrater.** The client is defensive, cautious, guarded, and constantly testing the counselor. They may want advice or solutions and expect the counselor to deliver. The client gets frustrated if they don't receive what they desire. The danger is that the counselor can provide easy solutions that don't encourage the client in taking responsibility and being accountable. There's a trap of seeing the client as more fragile than they are and doing for the client what they want instead of seeing this pattern as the root of transference.

5) **Counselor as non-entity.** The client regards the counselor as an inanimate figure without needs, wishes, desires, or problems. The client uses a barrage of words, doesn't listen to the counselor's interventions, and can create distance with outbursts. The counselor can feel overwhelmed and discounted.

Being aware of your own needs, motives, and personal reactions will help you focus on important therapeutic themes without getting side-tracked or confused while transference systems are operating. You will then be able to examine rather than react to the issues that are being transferred from the past into the present relationship with you. Be aware, however, that <u>not every</u> feeling a client has toward you is transference, i.e. if you've been rushed and not very present, your client may be justly disappointed, or if your client is angry with you, it may be justified and the relationship will need some attention.

Counter-transference[civ]

Counter-transference refers to the counselor's emotional reactions to the client, which may involve the counselor's own projections. These projections, e.g. the counselor's anxiety, need to be perfect, or need to control can get in the way of helping a client.

Constructive counter-transference can illuminate significant dynamics for the client. In destructive counter-transference, unresolved personal conflicts become entangled, and the counselor loses objectivity. This can become an ethical issue when the counselor uses the client to meet their own needs. The counselor can notice their own emotions as clues to unconscious motives of client, i.e. if the counselor becomes frustrated, it could be that the client is feeling anxious and wants progress to slow down.

Counter-transference patterns

Watson speaks of the problematic aspects of counter-transference patterns:

1) **Being overprotective of client.** A client can trigger the counselor's fears. The counselor then steers the client away from areas that trigger the counselor's painful material. The counselor softens remarks to protect from pain. The client is not challenged and thus avoids conflicts and struggles.

2) **Treating clients in benign ways.** The counselor has fears of the client's anger. To guard against this anger, the counselor creates superficiality and therapy degenerates into friendly conversation.

3) **Rejection of clients.** The counselor, seeing the client as needy and dependent, moves away, remains cool and aloof, and does not let the client get too close.

4) **Need for reinforcement and approval**. The counselor needs to be reassured of their effectiveness. If the client is not getting better, the counselor has fears and self-doubts.

5) **Seeing self in the client**. The counselor identifies with the client to the point of losing objectivity. They may see in the client traits

that the counselor dislikes in him or her self. A "difficult" client can be a mirror for the counselor.

6) **Development of sexual or romantic feelings.** The counselor can exploit the vulnerable position of the client, consciously or unconsciously. It is natural to be more attracted to some clients than to others. With awareness and sensitivity, feelings of attraction can be recognized, even acknowledged in a therapeutic relationship without becoming the focus of the therapy.

Examples of transference and counter-transference in action:

(a) Something a caregiver says unintentionally triggers memories of being treated disrespectfully in the past and client responds by withdrawing and shutting down as if the original disrespect were happening now.

(b) A client was wounded by sexual involvement with a former minister. When the new minister is warm and attentive, the client becomes convinced that new minister is making overt sexual overtures.

(c) A wife is angry at her husband but anger at him is not acceptable, so she gets angry at her caregiver.

(d) A client is convinced that the therapist is going to abandon him, when really the client is abandoning himself.

(e) When working with a particular client, a body worker often finds herself feeling incompetent, even though the client is satisfied. The therapist is projecting her past history with a critical teacher onto the client.

(f) A client reminds the therapist of his mother, and because he is not conscious of this association, he subtly and inappropriately projects these hostile, sexualized, or needy feelings onto the client.

(g) A counselor is so personally committed to her marriage that she fails to diagnose and treat spousal abuse in a couple she is working with.

Questions to ask yourself

Here are some questions to consider to increase your awareness about possible counter-transference issues that may need conscious attention:

- What am I feeling with this client?
- What do I want to say and do?
- What am I not saying?
- Do I find myself hoping this client won't come?
- Do I want this client to stay longer?

- Does this client remind me of someone else whom I am now having them be?
- Do I space out around this client?
- Do I have uncomfortable sensations in my body around this client?

Working with problematic transference

Once again, not all transferences cause difficulties, misunderstandings, or conflicts. Naming the situation is helpful and working with it directly can avoid escalation. A few suggestions:

- Name what you are noticing. "I'm noticing that whenever....... Are you aware of that too?"
- Be supportive, respectful, and non-judgmental with your client.
- Help your client discover and name who is in the background, historically. "Is this familiar somehow?"
- Explore how this transference is influencing the relationship, and how you might work with it.

Working with problematic counter-transference

- Be as alert as possible to distortions.
- Resolve it in yourself.
- Name this if this would be of therapeutic value.
- Get supervision, as needed.
- Make amends, if needed.

Working with problems includes paying attention to:

- projections
- transference
- counter-transference
- unconscious client/caregiver systems

Right use of power and influence involves understanding these basic notions and knowing that many conflicts arise from the distortions, misperceptions, and projections of both the client and the therapist. Many conflicts, misunderstandings, grievances, and lawsuits are founded in transference and counter-transference processes.

Self-Study Practice:

From the transference and counter-transference patterns described in this chapter, select one from each list that seems familiar to you. Reflect on

   a)   What are the indicators and how do you experience these transferences?
   b)   How do they affect your professional relationships?
   c)   Under what circumstances would it be necessary or useful to name and work with the transference?
   d)   What is the value and impact of working with the counter-transference in yourself?

Dimension Three: Be Connected

Topics covered in this section:
Impact & Intention
Boundaries
Supervision & Support
Resolving Difficulties
Grievance Processes
Referrals

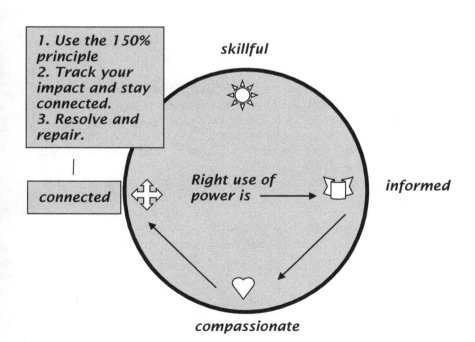

Focus on Connectedness
- *Right Use of Power depends on staying connected.*
- *Dimension Three is about Accountability.*
    - *Setting and maintaining boundaries*
    - *Understanding how grievance processes work*
    - *Being accountable for your relationships motivated by caring*
    - *Noticing (and responding non-defensively) when your impact doesn't match your intention*
    - *Making appropriate referrals*
    - *Getting supervision and support*
    - *Staying connected, resolving difficulties, and repairing the relationship*

Power Spiral—Topics in the Accountability Dimension

The direction for the connected and responsible use of power is in the West on the left side of the spiral.

Accountability is connected with healing, resolution, and self-correction. Accountability is best accompanied by caring, rather than guilt, force, or fear. The accountability dimension is devoted to helping caregivers integrate awareness about the power differential into caring and interactive responses. As one practitioner said, "I am now confident that I can use my power with love."

Accountability begins with non-defensively tracking for difficulties in the healing relationship. Caring use of power involves paying attention to impact when it doesn't match intention and attending to this impact within the relationship so that the conflict doesn't escalate beyond repair. This also involves determining when to let go, get help, or try another approach.

Being accountable for our behavior and caring about our impact on others brings deeper and more authentic relationships. Peace of mind and heart follow naturally.

In other chapters in this section, we explore boundaries as a centerpiece of accountable relationships. We also look at several kinds of grievance processes, guidelines for making referrals, and ways to use supervision.

Three Skills and Wisdoms

Use the 150% principle.

Let yourself be guided by the principle that although all parties bear responsibility (100%) for the health of the relationship, the one in the up-power role, has greater responsibility (150%). This helps balance responsibility with vulnerability and risk.

Track your impact and stay connected.

Staying connected depends on the ability to notice and be sensitive to clients' responses—both subtle and strong. Ethics is certainly about being connected and in right relationship. The power for health or for harm lies in the quality and integrity of the relationship.

Resolve and Repair

Staying connected, resolving difficulties, and repairing the relationship as soon as possible will usually prevent conflicts from escalating.

Barriers and Resources for Accountability

Working with the material in this section, participants have said such things as: "I see that I can get better at using difficulties to clarify, resolve, or deepen my connections, instead of avoiding conflict. It's a complete reframe on conflict." "I can be forgiven and be resourced by my goodness instead of my shame." "I need to allow myself to make mistakes, before I can allow others to."

Barriers to accountability often are accompanied by fear, shame, or paranoia. Beliefs such as "It's not my fault," "If I apologize for anything, it will be used against me." "They're making all this up," are reflected in habits of being defensive, accusing or blaming the other, not responding at all, hoping it will all go away on its own, or keeping secrets.

Resources include the power of right relatedness, ability to discern impacts and intentions, communication and problem solving skills, and ability to ask for support.

Power Spiral Layer

The power spiral layer associated with the West dimension could be considered the Power Spiral 4-step. It outlines four practices that support being in right relationship with your uses of both personal and role power.

4. Be Skillful

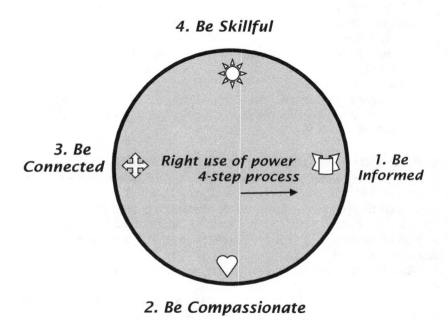

3. Be Connected

Right use of power 4-step process

1. Be Informed

2. Be Compassionate

Impact & Intention

Story: "Once at the end of a first session, my client asked for some "homework" so I suggested she do some journal writing about a habit she had discovered during the session. When she arrived for the next session, she sat down, looked at me, and immediately began almost screaming that she 'couldn't trust me...I was just like all the others...she knew this wasn't going to work...I had a formula that I applied to all my clients...and I wasn't going to take a personal interest in her...'. 'My goodness, you certainly have strong feelings!', I replied. 'Yes, I do! I just can't believe you gave me journal writing. I hate journal writing, and I bet you do that with everyone!' 'Well, I guess I've learned something about you. I'll never ask you to journal again!' She then burst out laughing at the absurdity of this much anger. Soon we were both laughing. I let her know I understood how important my personal attention and care were to her. She sat back and said, 'I can't tell you how touching it is that you are interested in learning about me and willing to change how you are in response. And, even more amazing that you didn't just reject me as a client.' My intention with journaling homework was to offer her something to think about and help her get more involved in therapy. The impact was that she felt distanced and uncared for. Her unconscious intention in her anger was to prove to herself that once again therapy wasn't going to help. The impact of my response was that she got treated the way she had longed for.*

Impact is the effect your behavior has on others. Intention is the effect you want to have.

The most effective and skillful use of power is made possible by being aware of and responsive to your impact on others. When your goal is to be of the best possible service to your clients, it is imperative to be interested in and attentive to their responses to your use of your Self, your role power, and your expertise. The best training and the best modalities will ultimately be compromised if you are not paying attention and then adjusting to how your clients are responding.

You may say one thing, for example, "I'd like to suggest you try…" but your impact may cause unexpected and unintended pain if your client takes this suggestion as a put down and manipulation. There need be no argument or defensiveness when this occurs, you and your client are both right. Your intention was good. Your client's experience (probably based on their past history) was of feeling misunderstood, judged, or disrespected. In other words, they felt harm.

Tracking and Housekeeping

Tracking is the moment to moment process of noticing your clients' responses to what is said, what they feel, the memories that emerge and the relationship itself. These responses will be visible or felt through tone of voice, postural movement, direct words, gestures and other physical manifestations. These can be quite subtle (for example, an emotion, if unnoticed and uncontacted disappears in a few seconds) or quite obvious changes in body language such as folding arms, looking away, tears.

By tracking for your impact, you can clarify and repair the relationship and prevent the difficulties from escalating. For example, you might say, "*I notice that you had quite a strong reaction to what I just said. I wonder if you understood what I said in a way I didn't intend.*" Clients let you know that they feel confused, misunderstood, or hurt. If you don't notice, they will keep letting you know in ways that become more exaggerated. **Good tracking skills are one of your best resources for preventing harm and repairing the relationship**.

Housekeeping is the process of keeping the relationship clear and productive. Just like houses, relationships need periodic cleaning—airing out, dusting, fixing a stuck window, water drip. It's no big deal, not good or bad, just some attention needed. If you break an egg on the floor, you clean it up. If there is a break or lack of clarity in the relationship, you clean it up-no big deal.[cv]

Examples of Impact differing from Intention

You may intend to support your client's independence, and your client may experience your support as rejection. *Your client's perceptions may be influenced by past history and therefore expectations of being abandoned may arise and bring feelings of rejection.*

You may intend warmth and compassion, and your client may experience this as pity. *Your client expects pity and therefore does not perceive compassion even when it is offered.*

Your client may intend to be clear about a boundary, and you may experience this as non-cooperation. *You may be concerned about being good enough, and therefore perceive every criticism as non-cooperation on the part of your client.*

You may intend comfort by a hand on your client's shoulder, and your client may respond as if you were a former abuser. *Your client may transfer feelings, responses, or expectations onto you that belong to someone else in their life.*

You may intend respect, and your client experiences disrespect. *The meaning of direct eye contact differs in your client's culture.*

Misperceptions of intention can occur on the part of either the caregiver or the client. Unintended impacts happen consistently in organizations as well. *Story: An organization had a policy for resolving interpersonal conflicts within the organization. Step 1: try to resolve personally, Step 2: bring in a third party, Step 3: take the conflict to your supervisor. This is a common recommendation based in trying to empower people to work out their issues themselves rather than always bringing them to an up-power person. However, the Director of the agency discovered that there were many conflicts that never got resolved and just went underground. In consulting with me, the Director understood that, in fact, his employees felt ashamed and incompetent when they couldn't resolve a conflict interpersonally and also didn't want to risk their performance evaluation by bringing the conflict to a supervisor. This was definitely an unintended consequence. The resolution was for the Director to create a confidential "care and repair" team who were empowered to offer employees coaching, support, a listening ear, and, in addition, mediation services when needed. As a result, employees felt supported and resourced rather than punished or at risk.*

In human beings, past experiences often become beliefs that then become embodied as self-protective strategies. These strategies then become expectations about how they will be treated. People often have different experiences of the same event, because we all bring our own history and expectations to every relationship.

Power Differential Impact

Story: Therapist expresses appreciation of some progress that has been made. Client reacts with anger and resentment at this "insincerity" because he is transferring his feelings from an argument he just had with his girlfriend.

In professional relationships, the power differential increases the potential for difference between impact and intention. Cultural, sexual, religious, and class differences strongly influence discrepancies between intention and impact. *(Refer to the chapter on transference and counter-transference for more about how transference can affect impact.)*

A lack of understanding of this very simple concept of intention and impact accounts for a surprisingly large percentage of relationship difficulties. When you know your intention to be good, it can be challenging to shift your perspective to understand that your client experiences these actions and words as painful, critical, disrespectful, or confusing. When you understand that both of you are "right" in being true to your experience of a set of words or a behavior, resolution no longer needs to be focused on who's wrong, but rather, about clarifying how you understood each other.

Understanding the difference between intention and impact can help you shift your focus from defending your position to one of curiosity; from who is right or wrong to clarifying intentions; from anger to compassion; and from giving up to resolution and relationship repair.

Keep in mind that your client may have a hard time standing up for him or herself because of the impact of the power differential. Your client may withdraw, swallow feelings, take their distress elsewhere, or their feelings may come out in other ways. It may be challenging to learn how to handle misunderstandings with grace, immediacy, and non-defensiveness.

Five Keys

You may find these keys useful for unlocking impact and intention discrepancies. In resolving and getting reconnected, what's most important is not what you meant but understanding how it was received.

Sensitize yourself to the possibility that your impact was different from your intention.

Listen to your client's experience. *(i.e. "Please tell me about your experience just now.)*

Validate your client's experience. *(i.e. "I can understand how you could feel [hurt]."")*

Explain your intention in a simple way. (*i.e. "It wasn't my intention to hurt you. My intention was _____.)*

Ask what else is needed. (i.e., *"How are you feeling now?"* Or, *"Is there anything else you need around this?"* Or, *"How are we doing now? Is there anything needed for relationship repair?"* *"What I wish I had don/said is . . . . and what I'll do next time is . . . ."*)

Tracking and contacting impact can help the relationship self-correct quickly and successfully. Like navigating a sailboat, the person at the helm keeps the goal in sight but uses the wind to tack and then correct. The journey seldom takes one straight line to the dot on the horizon, but the more frequently you self-correct, the smoother and quicker your arrival. A big self-correction takes a lot more effort than a little one, but too many tiny corrections can slow the process to a snail's pace.

Self-Study: Responding to impact

1. Make a little list of examples of impact being different from intention.

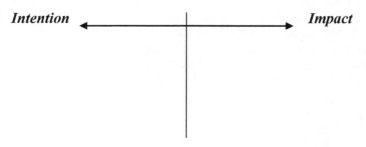

2. Now recall a time in your professional experience when your impact was different from your intention and didn't turn out well.

What happened?
How did you feel?
What was the result?

3. Now, in your imagination, replay the event (making written notes, or role-playing it with a partner), trying out responding using the five steps that have been outlined.

Sensitize
Listen
Validate
Explain
Ask

4. What do you imagine would be different in the result?

Boundaries

"The task is to recognize our interdependence, honor boundaries and differences, and remember connectedness."

— *Dyrian Benz[cvi]*

"Find the optimum closeness/distance to enable you to experience your OWN unique center of aliveness and awareness, as well as the other's unique center."

— *Mukara Meredith[cvii]*

Good boundaries are a centerpiece for safe and successful relationships.

Boundaries are, as well, the space that people consider part of their identity. Skin is the physical boundary. People also have energetic and emotional boundaries. Inadvertent boundary crossings can be very upsetting. Boundaries are very individual, can be negotiated between people, and are often communicated non-verbally. They are influenced by cultural values, styles and expectations. Try checking with your clients about precisely what feels to them like the right distance from you. You may be surprised about the amount of variation. After several sessions in which I sat my usual distance, I noticed a slight holding back and asked my client about it. I was surprised to discover that, for her, the truly safe distance was five feet away! Starting at the safe distance of five feet, we were able in a few more sessions work with her self-protection issues enough for her to feel safe at a closer distance. Boundaries serve well to provide a consistent container that can define, contain, and limit relationships.

Development of Boundaries

The development of boundaries is a strong aspect of individuation. Boundaries are a fundamental aspect of self-development. Infants are born into a swirling world of new and familiar sensations in which they experience no distinction between self and other—all are merged into one. This is the beginning of the universal and lifelong process of finding a Self. Boundaries define and protect. They allow separation and they can be negotiated to experience the joy of merging. They can provide both freedom and protection.

Healthy boundary development proceeds through stages briefly described by my colleague Mukara Meredith[cviii] as:

1) "Undifferentiated" with the developmental need being to feel welcome and secure in the containment of the caretaker.

2) "Separate but Surrounded" with the developmental need being support and nourishment.

3) "Open Support" with the need for developing autonomy by coming and going from caretaker's protective presence.

4) "Overlapping" with the need to be able to say no and still belong.

5) "Individuated" with the need to join and separate, and be creative and unique, without fear of loss of love.

Boundary Styles

To various degrees in our self-development, all of us, both clients and helping professionals have experienced challenges and wounds. Therefore, we adopt boundary styles that, although designed to be protective, actually may limit relationship satisfaction.

Relationship-limiting styles include over-bounded, under-bounded, and pendulum styles. Experientially, **over-bounded** is an "automatic no" style. Relationships are compromised because there is no way to get close. As Bradshaw[cix] says, "there's no door knob to the self." Those with this boundary style have difficulty letting go, softening, nourishing or being nourished. They over-protect out of such potent fear of being hurt that they are out of touch with Self's ability to be resilient and appropriately protective. Experientially, **under-bounded** is an "automatic yes" style. Relationships are compromised because there is little sense of the other. Good relationships actually *thrive* in the interface of differences. Users of this style feel so frightened of being abandoned, that they lose touch with Self and they have created the illusionary belief that there will then be nothing to reject. They feel vague, confused about what they want and need, and try to merge with others. Those who use the **pendulum style** flip back and forth from over-bounded to under-bounded. This style compromises relationship by being unpredictable.

Effective boundaries are both secure and flexible. Saying "no" is the simplest form of boundary setting, and may, at times, be necessary to forcefully exert for the protection of clients and others from harm. As a practitioner, you need to be sensitive and responsive to your client's boundaries, knowing that they may be different from yours. You can increase your sensitivity to your clients' boundary styles and concerns by understanding your own style and how it is likely to impact your clients.

Self-Study Practices

1. Boundary habits

Take a moment to self-reflect on your boundary habits. Where do you tend to land in terms of these continuums:

Over-bounded ----------------------------	Under-bounded
Not enough differentiation ----------------------------	Not enough integration
Inflexible ----------------------------	Elusive
Controlling ----------------------------	Easily controlled
Rigid ----------------------------	Merged
Uncompromising ----------------------------	Vague and confused

Imagine what kinds of confusion, misunderstanding, or difficulties could arise when you, as a professional with a tendency to be inflexible with boundaries, try to work with a client whose boundaries tend to be elusive.

2. The 150% principle with boundaries

As the person in the position of greater power and influence, it is your responsibility to set and maintain boundaries. Even though your clients agree to the boundaries you set and often help you in creating the boundaries, you are ultimately responsible for the boundaries. The 150% principle applies. These are the basic boundaries.

• *Physical*	• *Emotional*
• *Mental*	• *Energetic*
• *Sexual*	• *Financial*
• *Environmental*	• *Social*
• *Time*	• *Role*

Here are some boundary examples in which the power differential can have a significant and harmful impact:

Physical: using touch unconsciously or not attending to spatial boundaries

Emotional: encouraging emotional dependence or being too personally revealing so that your clients feel they must take care of you

Mental: creating a psychologically impactful "smart/dumb" dynamic

Energetic: communicating through one's energy a more intimate relationship than is real or appropriate

Sexual: becoming intimately involved with your client or encouraging or implying the possibility

Financial: not being clear about your financial contracting or keeping a client longer than they are benefiting from your service

Environmental: not creating a safe, private, and attractive office setting

Social: engaging in or not managing dual relationships

Time: not holding clear time boundaries by being late or going over the time, rushing or being abrupt, or not having or keeping a clear cancellation policy

Role: not owning and skillfully using the power you have

Take a few minutes to reflect on each of these professional boundaries and notice how you are in relation to each one on the continuum of 1 (not so good) to 10 (fine).

Physical	⊢————————————————→	10
Emotional	⊢————————————————→	10
Mental	⊢————————————————→	10
Energetic	⊢————————————————→	10
Sexual	⊢————————————————→	10
Financial	⊢————————————————→	10
Environmental	⊢————————————————→	10
Social	⊢————————————————→	10
Time	⊢————————————————→	10
Role	⊢————————————————→	10

Pick one of these to work on handling better. Choose a specific and behavioral way you can make some improvement. Arrange to get some feedback from a friend or colleague.

3. Checklists
a. Boundary checklist

Joanna Colrain and Kathy Steele[cx] offer these topics for use in initial meetings. Which ones do you use and/or need?

- educational credentials
- time parameters for session
- fee structure
- cancellation policy
- availability by phone or in emergency
- confidentiality agreement and exceptions
- termination
- terms required by insurance providers
- supervision
- entitlement to second opinion at any time
- sexual touch or intimacy is unethical
- grievance process
- records
- method of therapy and techniques used as requested by client
- other (particular to your modality)
- disclosure form

b. Professional limits

Here are some questions from Colrain and Steele to consider in relation to your boundaries.

- What kinds of clients do you take and how many of them?
- How do you decide a client is too difficult or complex to work with?
- What types of clients will you *NOT* work with?
- Are you willing to go over your client limit for clients in crisis?
- Do you work weekends and/or holidays? Do you take vacations? Do you take calls on vacation?
- How comfortable are you saying "no?"
- Do you start and end sessions on time?
- What is your comfort level with your personal boundaries and limits?
- How can you tell if you are within your limits or have overstepped them?
- What are your particular signs of stress or burnout?

c. Personal Limits

Also from Colrain and Steele: what are your personal limits around:

- Physical contact
- Phone calls
- Extended sessions
- Giving personal information
- Therapy outside the office
- Community contact
- Contact with the family
- Grounds for termination
- Gift-giving
- Receiving fees
- Clients who owe you money
- Amount of credit you will extend and length of time

Supervision & Support

"Working without supervision or a review process, mistakes stay internalized and never talked about. But in a practice where 'everything' is out in the open, potential and actual problems are quickly and compassionately dealt with and learned from. It is wrong to think you can surface and take care of any ethical situation by yourself," writes a student.

When was the last time you talked with a colleague or supervisor about an ethical issue, dilemma, or mistake? In using your power to prevent and reduce harm, supervision and peer support are some of your best allies. Reluctance to use supervision and support for ethical concerns has several very natural and understandable sources:

- Shame leading to silence
- Embarrassment about an action or feeling
- Fear of consequences or punishment
- Lack of awareness of an ethical issue
- Unwillingness to acknowledge harm

Talking with a supervisor about an ethical concern takes courage, integrity, and a desire to be accountable. The level of challenge or vulnerability experienced or anticipated by most professionals increases in the following progression:

      6. legal action
     5. unresolved situation in which you misused power
    4. currently escalating situation
   3. current dilemma
  2. resolved situation in which you caused harm
 1. engaging in a role play of an ethical issue

Here are several stories:

• *Susan as a bodyworker prided herself in her good boundaries. However, as a single person very interested in partnership, when she found herself apparently mutually attracted to one of her clients, she lost her perspective. As she said, "My hands grow bigger, and my mind grows smaller, when love is before me." She found herself fantasizing about getting into a relationship with this client. Surprised by the strength of her thoughts, she sought supervision. Heeding the honest feedback from her supervisor helped deal with her feelings and stay in right relationship.*

• *Mark was a new therapist and in wanting to build his practice and make his services affordable, he had agreed to trade therapy for housecleaning. However, his client seemed resentful about working for a lower hourly rate than Mark was working and was doing a slow and inadequate job. Mark was embarrassed that from his need for work, he had agreed on such a trade, but by being willing to talk with his supervisor about it, they were able to figure out a plan to reduce the harm. Mark would tell his client that he had mistakenly agreed to the trade which created a dual role relationship that was not an ethical situation, apologize for the awkwardness, and ask his client to instead volunteer his time with a service group of his choice.*

• *Nancy talked about each of her clients in supervision. She was particularly pleased about her work with one of her clients since this client repeatedly told Nancy that she was the best therapist she'd ever had and how helpful and important therapy was to her. Over time, her supervisor, began to notice that even though this client was pleased, they weren't doing much deep or effective work. When she brought this observation to Nancy's attention, it became clear to Nancy that she had, through her client's praise, begun to collude with her client to not really look at the painful issues she had come to therapy to work on. Getting caught in a system is something that happens often in helping relationships and is hard to see without outside help.*

• *Bill was most surprised when one of his former clients filed an ethical grievance for being abandoned. He had kept records about the termination process and also informed his supervisor of the appropriate steps he had taken. These records were the evidence needed for the case to be dismissed.*

Supervision Relationship dynamics arising from:
• the power differential
• transference and counter-transference

- diversity issues
- system-based expectations and responsibilities

are often complex and outside conscious awareness and can, when not noticed and attended to, result in harm to clients.

Support is available from a number of sources, including professional supervision, peer support groups, and continuing education courses.

When ethical dilemmas or errors happen, wise and skillful attention is needed immediately to prevent escalation beyond repair. Therefore, it is vital to have appropriate and adequate supervision in place before a problem emerges. The impulse to avoid the situation by not bringing it up at all, minimizing, blaming your client, and/or hoping it will just go away is strong. Supervision can bring perspective back.

Seeking Guidance

Supervision and support situations in which there are safety, compassion, honesty, trust, and integrity are most helpful. Whether you have an assigned supervisor or the freedom to choose one, ask a few questions in advance to find out how he or she feels about ethical issues. Ask yourself what you need to feel safe enough to be truthful and vulnerable about ethical issues. Ask them about their perspective, their approach to conflict resolution and repair of harm, and the kind of help they can offer you.

Supervision and peer support that focuses on honest self-assessment, self-correction, repair and re-education will be most beneficial. Arrange for support and use it wisely. In situations where you can choose your supervisor and/or peer support, include these considerations in your choices.

- Do you respect this person?
- Are they compassionate and trustworthy?
- Do they have good boundaries and keep confidentiality?
- Is it safe to be truthful and vulnerable?

In summary, peer support and professional supervision offer essential opportunities for...

- feedback about impact
- accurate self-assessment
- emotional support
- outside perspective
- problem-solving

- acknowledgement and encouragement

Good supervision can prevent and reduce harm from ethical mistakes both to yourself and your clients, protect you from false accusations and help you learn from and not repeat errors.

Here's an example of using supervision to guide you in a sensitive situation, keeping the best interests of your client as the highest priority. Ira Byock, a well-known physician who focuses on palliative care for patients who are dying, talks here about his relationship with Sharon, a teenager with multiple life-threatening conditions that were not improving through the available treatments. With caring and skillful attention, Dr. Byock gained Sharon's trust. Over time, to bring a little brightness to a bleak hospital life, he arranged to take Sharon on brief trips outside the hospital--out to lunch, to a pet store because Sharon loved animals, to an ice cream shop. At a staff meeting, a social worker on Dr. Byock's team honestly brought up the question about whether his giving Sharon such special attention was ethical.

Dr. Byock replied, *"I took the matter seriously, but not from a lack of confidence in the propriety of my actions. . . . Our team used our regular weekly education meetings to discuss these issues. Professional boundaries serve to protect vulnerable patients from manipulative doctors. But clear professional boundaries also free physicians and patients to be authentic with one another. We had lively discussions and came to the conclusion that befriending people who happen to be our patients is not a transgression. Whenever possible, we decided we should pamper our patients. . . . 'Sometimes it's okay to take a kid to a pet store.' Far from representing a violation of professional boundaries, I felt it was a privilege to help Sharon. I made her life a little better in simple ways, by truly caring for her. It would have been inauthentic to suppress the impulse to do so."* [cxi] Regular staff meetings such as this promote ongoing dialogue and increased sensitivity to issues, especially those with shades of gray.

Resourcing Yourself through Internet Technology

The internet and smartphones are now primary communication tools and have become an essential part of work, daily contacts, networking and marketing. They have also become a major source of stress, distraction, misinformation, addiction, lowered self-esteem, and decreased empathy. Email, for example, can increase stress because every email arrives in the in-box looking the same--same format, same size font--thus seeming equally urgent. Email messages are notoriously easily misinterpreted.

When we send an email we literally don't see the impact on the receiver and so can't respond appropriately and right away. As my friend Christine Hart puts it, "Mass media has a disease of disempathy with the nervous system." We can say anything we want and not be connected to the feedback loop of in-person contact. Further, email cc- lists keep us in an enormous number of communication loops that we need not be involved in. It is so easy to get "sucked in" and addicted to Facebook and checking e-mails.

Right use of technology means using technology to serve your needs, rather than putting technology in the driver's seat. Easier said than done. We have a lot to learn. For starters, here are a few strategies you might try. Set a timer and only do email for this set amount of time. Take one day a week off from all email communication. Set specific times of the day (maybe 3) to check email. Also decide on certain times and amounts of time to use Facebook. Decide on times and places when you will not use your smartphone.

The world-wide-web is a major resource for information about virtually any question or concern. Internet research is, in fact, one of the most useful and time-saving ways to get up-to-date information on specific ethical issues and professional dialogues. Computer technology has exponentially increased our access to relationships and information in all realms. Technology has likely changed our brains and our nervous systems. Like most neutral things, use of technology needs to be guided by moral values, self-care, choice, and spaciousness. Like most neutral things, we need to use technology wisely and well, and not be enslaved or depraved by it.

> *"Out beyond our ideas of right doing and wrong doing is a field. I'll meet you there."* —*Rumi*[cxii]

Self-Study: Accessing Guidance

Choose a personal ethical situation—a current dilemma, or a past mistake—and then, using discernment questions, choose a supervisor or colleague to talk with (or imagine talking with) about this. What do you need to feel safe enough to be truthful? Notice your level of vulnerability or shame. Acknowledge what you learn from this process.

What I need to be truthful
    1.
    2.
    3.
Level of vulnerability and/or shame in talking about this.

1 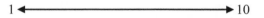 10

What I learned
    1.
    2.
    3.

What I will do differently now.
    1.

Resolving Difficulties

The phone message said, "I want to come in for a completion session because I need to use my financial resources for something else." Steven, a body psychotherapist, wondered what else might be going on for this client who had not yet met the goals she had set for herself. When Carrie came for her completion session, she focused on how great therapy had been and how thankful she was, and how unfortunately she just couldn't afford to come anymore. Steven sensed some other energy and asked Carrie, "Is there anything at all that you are disappointed about?" Carrie answered, "No, you have been such a good listener and so patient and insightful." Steven checked again. "Thank you. As I think about the work we've done together, I wonder if you feel discouraged that the problem you came in to work on hasn't resolved even though you've gotten clearer about it?"

Carrie was silent for a time and then, apparently feeling safe and encouraged, took what was a big risk for her. She spoke thoughtfully. "Yes, actually, I am disappointed. I've done a lot of therapy and once again it seems like it hasn't worked. If it was working, I'd feel like my money was being well-used." Steven contacted her feelings and courage and thanked her for being so honest. Carrie went on. "And something else, I have felt a little uncomfortable with how close to me you move your chair, and sometimes, like when we did the experiment when we were pushing hands so I could find out about anger, touching was too much. But I thought, you're the therapist and I really want to change and so I never said anything."

Steven took a breath and responded. "Thank you for telling me. Again that must have taken courage. I am so sorry that I wasn't tracking the cues you have given me about your discomfort. Could we spend a few minutes with this? I'll start moving my chair back and you tell me when the distance feels just right." After finding and experiencing the right distance, which turned out to be about six feet away, Steven suggested an experiment in awareness in which he would move slowly closer. She would hold up her hand when she began to feel uncomfortable and they could both notice what happened. Steven described tracking a slight tensing in her cheeks, but otherwise, everything about Carrie's demeanor and posture seemed visibly unchanged to him when she was uncomfortable.

Carrie had an insight: "I feel it all inside me and I put a lot of effort into making sure that you won't notice anything that might not be agreeable." Steven responded: "Great insight. So, it seems that you have been working hard for me not to be able to notice. And you succeeded, but it cost you a lot of suffering. I'm imagining you might be a bit angry that I didn't notice." "Well, yes. You're the therapist. You're supposed to notice. I don't want to have to tell you. Then I feel like I'm doing your job!" From this interaction, Steven was able to self-correct by being more attuned to Carrie's discomfort cues and her fears of not being liked. Carrie had had a successful experience of revealing discomfort and not being rejected. She took a several month break. and then returned to work successfully, this time, being more personally engaged and self-disclosing in her relationships. Had Steven not found a way to help Carrie talk about these concerns, her sense of betrayal and distrust could have escalated into a grievance.

Understanding and abiding by ethical codes, laws, and grievance processes is essential. Ethics can and must also be relationship-prudent. Right Use of Power ethics is relational. Motivated by caring and compassion, ethical awareness and actions are finely tuned to relationships and relationship concerns. Relationship-prudence is a good term for ethical behavior guided by consideration of the best interests of clients, students and others in down-power roles.

No matter how good our intentions, we make mistakes, we have a complex impact on others, we misunderstand power dynamics, we are naïve, we project and are projected on, we cause harm. When acknowledged and attended to, most mistakes can be corrected and most harm can be repaired. A number of studies have shown that what people need when they have been harmed in a helping relationship is surprisingly simple: acknowledgment of their experience, clarification about how it happened, an apology or regret, and assurance that the same thing won't happen again.

"Life is a great teacher—first you get the experience, and then you get the lesson."[cxiii] We, as caregivers, have an enormous capacity to learn and self-correct. Relationship-prudence focuses on reducing and repairing harm that, in turn, can clarify and resolve relationship difficulties, deepen trust and understanding, and model successful resolution of conflict. Relationship-prudence can help avoid litigation and grievance actions.

Take a minute now to remember and reflect on what motivated and inspired you to become a helping professional. Acknowledge and honor your altruism and desire to serve.

Ultimately, global survival depends on our ability to resolve conflicts peacefully and for the greater good. Peaceful resolution of conflict is a high art and skill. There are exceptional books, programs, and resources available on this topic. Faith, intention, and practice in resolving difficulties within your professional relationships supports many positive outcomes. It will prevent grievances; clarify, repair, and deepen client relationships; model staying connected through conflict; and seed confidence in the human ability to resolve conflict peacefully in other contexts.

Whether or not a conflict is resolved successfully is significantly impacted by three factors on the part of the caregiver. The caregiver, as the up-power person, bears 150% of the responsibility for tracking and attending to the difficulty. Tracking with curiosity, non-defensiveness, and empathy are the primary skills to develop.

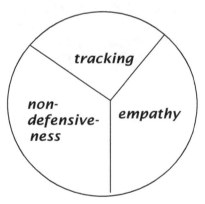

Escalation of conflict or disconnect

Conflicts seek resolution. Sometimes the difficulty is more of a relationship-disconnect than a conflict. Disconnects also seek reconnection. When conflict, disconnects, and misunderstandings arise with clients, they tend to escalate very quickly and dramatically, often out of proportion to the situation.

Story: A therapist, acting ethically, concluded that he needed to refer his client to someone else because his client's issues were beyond the scope of his training. His client felt rejected and because the therapist didn't notice and contact his client's response during their last session, the situation escalated to an ethics complaint claiming abandonment. The grievance process to ascertain responsibility and deal with the harm was lengthy, expensive, and time consuming. In this case, the conflict could have been resolved by a prompt, non-defensive response acknowledging his client's feelings. In this example, the therapist lacked the three skills most important to resolving problems: tracking, non-defensiveness and empathy.

Tracking for and attending to conflict in its initial stage is one of the most important skills for staying in right relationship, and for preventing ethical grievances. Here is a set of skills that can lead to amicable resolutions.

First Skill—Tracking Indicators

The first skill to develop is the ability to track for indicators of a problem. Clients will let you know in many ways, some subtle and some obvious, that they are having difficulty with you. Clients' felt experience of difficulty usually begins with feeling rejected, disliked, taken advantage of, disrespected, dismissed, over-powered, or unsafe. When these feelings are not recognized and acknowledged, they escalate.

Here are some indicators that the relationship may need attention:

Expressive Indicators
- making a direct statement of concern, fear, or anger
- showing posture, body, or facial signals of distress or concern
- asking for reassurance
- showing frustration
- showing general or consistent sense of confusion
- a change in breathing rhythm
- fidgeting
- processing in a repetitive way
- client or practitioner consistently feeling depleted or bored

Contractive Indicators
- canceling, being late, or failing to keep appointment
- deflecting input
- disguising a concern in a question
- disconnecting emotionally, withdrawing, or shutting down
- exhibiting a discrepancy between words and body
- acting too polite, compliant, or reassuring

- showing tension or tightening
- showing stillness or frozenness
- making no or little eye contact
- the session feeling stuck
- increasing dependency and disempowerment
- showing coldness or aloofness

Internal Indicators

- any of the above that you notice in yourself
- a thought or felt sense of something being "off"
- feeling triggered
- recognizing a familiar habit or system
- noticing counter-transference

Second Skill—Empathy

Upon tracking an indicator of a relationship problem, disconnect or difficulty, shift your focus toward what you are noticing. Engage your curiosity. Contact your client's experience directly, letting him or her know you are interested and concerned. The sooner you recognize and attend to conflict, the less likely a conflict will escalate.

Third Skill—Non-defensiveness

Responding non-defensively is easier said than done. For most people, conflict is hooked up with loss, pain, blame, and often trauma. Naturally, we want to defend ourselves or avoid the conflict. Non-defensiveness requires consciously reversing habitual patterns of avoiding conflict. Lack of experience and skill in peacefully and successfully resolving conflict and repairing relationships is a chronic global problem. So, what to do? First, look at this list of conflict-avoiding strategies and identify the ones that you use. Then try to connect to your hope and confidence that problems can be resolved. One of the simplest and most effective shifts is moving from defensiveness to curiosity. In my classes, people pair up and imagine a relational conflict between them. They notice their habitual responses. Then they close their eyes and change only one thing: they engage their curiosity. They then open their eyes and notice what changes. They report things like: "It's now less about the conflict and more about the relationship; and, I'm less tense and more hopeful."

Conflict-avoiding strategies include:
- over-analyzing
- shifting the blame
- shutting down and withdrawing
- taking all the blame or over-apologizing
- minimizing or exaggerating
- crying
- defending good intentions
- denying, pretending or ignoring the problem
- taking it out on someone else
- agreeing about everything
- making a joke
- rationalizing
- proactive, dismissive understanding
- self-righteousness

The fact that you have a conflict or difficulty with a client or they have perceived you as causing them harm does not in itself determine that you are unethical or guilty. It means that the relationship and the situation need immediate attention. The practice of reframing conflict as an event or process that can be used positively is helpful. Turning toward conflict with a stated and hopeful intention of resolution is truly ethical behavior.

Resolving and Repairing
When people feel they have been wounded or mistreated, they usually need remarkably simple things. Referring to the following chart, your client may often need just the first thing (empathy), or they may need any or all of the additional pieces. Track for indicators that the situation is resolved. You don't need to make a bigger deal than it is. Discern when you've done enough and stop there.

What clients need (any or all of these)

1. ACKNOWLEDGEMENT
They want their experience acknowledged, understood, validated, and empathized. They want to be appreciated for their willingness to talk about this feeling or issue.

2. UNDERSTANDING
They may want to know what happened, or what your intention was, if there is a difference between your intention and the impact.

3. APOLOGY OR REGRET
They want a genuine apology or expression of regret.
Apology form*: 1) This is what (my behavior) I regret. . . .
   2) This is what I am doing to make sure it doesn't happen again. . .
   3) Is there anything you need from me right now about this?
Regret form: (examples) "I'm sorry that we have gotten disconnected over something that wasn't in my awareness." "I'm sorry that I didn't hear you correctly." "I regret that I hurt you by not acknowledging what you said."

4. LEARNING
They want reassurance that you've learned or understood something about yourself or how to better care for them, and that you will act differently in the future.

5. REPAIR
They want to reconnect and participate in repair of the relationship or in gaining clarity and letting go.

* from Magi Cooper

Studies show that people, if they are treated in the above manner, will be far less likely to file a grievance or law suit and will have increased trust and satisfaction as a client when a problem has been successfully resolved.

Resolving Conflict and/or
Addressing Misuse of Power with Superiors

What about resolving difficulties with superiors? Since the power difference is role-dependent, you will find yourself in roles on both sides of the differential. You may go from seeing a client in your office (in your up-power role) to talking with your supervisor (in your down-power role). In fact, we move between up-power and down-power positions multiple times in a day. For example, you may go from being a patient at the doctor's office to being a supervisor to being a supervisee to being an employer to being an employee to being a driver encountering a policeman. Moving between up-power and down-power roles requires a shift in context and way of being with power. The amount of this shift varies by situation.

Trying to resolve conflict, asking for changes, and/or addressing misuses of power with superiors takes more skill, sensitivity, and resilience than working with these things with those down-power to you. While the five things listed as needed by clients could be useful with superiors, there are other things that will be helpful when resolving things using down-power influence. For example, be skillful, be strategic, be kind, link a complaint with a specific request for change, find and use the places you have leverage, give specific examples, be willing to negotiate, be simple/consistent/persistent, have courage in the face of authority, try to understand even though you don't agree, stay calm. See more about using down-power influence in the chapters on Leadership and Soul Work and World Service.

Here is a model from Cornelius and Faire[cxiv] that also has five elements and has been found to be effective in working things out with a superior. Try it with a relatively simple and straightforward issue before addressing something more complex. See page 291-295 for additional suggestions.

What superiors may need to respond well to your initiatives.

1. *ACTION OR EVENT*
   Say what happened without loading the description with emotive words.

2. *YOUR RESPONSE*
   Say how you feel or how it affected you without blame. You may also want to explain why you feel that way.

3. *PREFERRED OUTCOME*
   Say what you'd like to be able to do or have, or simply: "I'd like to work something out together." No demands. Make it an invitation.

4. *CONSTRUCTIVE CONSEQUENCE*
   Describe the benefit(s) to the relationship and/or the job of the outcome you are suggesting. Try to enroll your superior.

5. *INVITATION TO RESPOND*
   Encourage a conversation.

Story: Maggie was feeling increasingly frustrated and marginalized. Part of her job was to develop a handbook for her co-workers about resources for dealing with crises. Every time she asked for feedback and support, her supervisor told her she had other things to work on and was sure Maggie was doing fine. Maggie tried the process above: "When I don't get specific feedback on how I am designing and writing this project, I feel unsure, unimportant, and I lose motivation to keep working. I'd like to sit down with you and look at it together. This would improve both the project and my energy and motivation for completing it. When could we make some time? I think half an hour would be enough." Maggie was surprised when her supervisor quickly made the time and the handbook was soon completed. Maggie's supervisor volunteered that what had been most effective for her was hearing from Maggie that only half an hour was needed, how this request would be of benefit, and not being criticized for putting her off several times.

1. The Power of Empathy

Empathy is a powerful offering. With empathy, you can simply ask the other person to describe their complaint about you. While the other person explains, listen intently, and then say, as Bill Reidler [cxv] outlines, *"When I do that (give a brief but accurate description of their complaint using their words, followed by an example of when you did what they are complaining about.) I must make you feel_____." (Feel the feelings while you are saying this. Deeply empathize.) Make sure the complaining person feels heard, understood, and feels like his complaint is a valid complaint. Now I am aware that this sounds overly simplistic. But it really works! It will take a lot of practice to develop the ability to sincerely empathize. And it will be difficult to avoid defending and to stifle the urge to blame the other party. But if we make the investment in practicing and learning empathy, it will melt the majority of conflicts.* The miracle of compassionate understanding brings a "softening" of the energy around an issue. Often, this is enough.

2. The Power of Truth

There are two major mistakes in responding to conflicts and misunderstandings: **A) Taking it ALL personally, and B) taking NONE of it personally.** People commonly fear that if they take accusations or conflict personally, they will end up being attacked even more or end up with all the responsibility on their shoulders. "If I soften up, I'll get hurt and I won't be able to protect myself." So how can we be open to the truth in the complaint and not end with all the blame?

There is often some combination of truth and projection when relationship difficulties arise. It is important to take your client's feedback sincerely and personally, and to understand that the difficulty will also be reflecting personal history and habits. There is almost always a germ of personal truth. Part of acknowledging your client's experience and sharing your intention is to own and clarify that truth. Once your client's experience has been acknowledged and validated, you can use this clarity to go deeper. In addition, by empathizing, you model what it is like to be self-accepting. We all need to develop self-acceptance so that we are willing to see what mistakes we have made that inadvertently cause others to be angry with us. This self-acceptance makes it easier for your client to comfortably recognize if or how he or she has participated in the problem.

3. The Power of Compassion and Curiosity

Your client needs to know you care and to experience your compassion. An appropriate apology or expression of sorrow for their experience can be very simply stated. No need to go into long explanations that end up focusing the attention on you.

Compassion is the ability to feel another's suffering as both different from your own and connected to your own—suffering as universal experience and as inspiration for your desire to connect and help. Within the arms of compassion, resolving relationship difficulties is an expression of care, integrity, and confidence rather than an action coming out of fear of punishment.

Compassion accompanied by curiosity profoundly shifts the energy by softening hearts and re-focusing on inquiry rather than blame or judgment. Curiosity is a quality that builds connection and collaboration.

4. The Power of Moan and Groan

Having a safe and confidential place to air your feelings and thoughts without having to make them acceptable or kind, helps create internal spaciousness and relief. When someone, even a client, steps on your toes, you need a place to say "ouch." If the feelings are anger, you may find a piece of wisdom about your boundaries or needs that could help you work with the boundaries and needs of your clients. From a clear space, skillfulness is easier to access and use. A supervisor, colleague, or friend can provide this kind of place.

5. The Power of Apology

Authentic and effective apology is the very core of healing, clarifying and restoring relationships across a broad range of situations from interpersonal to organizational to cross-cultural. A real and well-thought-out apology can, like forgiveness, cut the cycle of anger, revenge, and hatred. However, making a genuine apology causes the giver to be extremely vulnerable. You are admitting directly to another that you did something that caused them harm. This is humbling. Apologizing is also challenging because it's like leaping off a cliff into the unknown. You are not in charge of how your apology will be received. Your efforts could be harshly rejected. *Story: Through psychotherapy, Alan, an M.D., understood that his efforts at friendship with a distressed client were inappropriate, and were experienced as a sexual come-on. His first apology was poorly received. Here's how it went: "I'm sorry you felt hurt, but you made it up. I was not coming on to you." He made very common mistakes: being defensive, making her wrong, not taking any responsibility for his behavior, and not offering either apology or repair. His second attempt was much better but was still rejected. He was left with a big lesson.*   There are many reasons that even skillful apologies may be rejected. These have to do with the wounded person's ability to be receptive. Even so, skillful apology is worth the effort.

On the other hand, your efforts could, and more likely will, be gratefully received and lead to some deep healing and relationship repair. *Story: In a class that I was supervising taught by a new teacher, one of the students shared an experience and insight she had had during a classroom practice time. The teacher responded in a way that seemed to indicate that she had not understood the student. I made note of this in order to give her feedback later. In a few minutes the same thing happened again. This time the student said, "That isn't at all what I was saying." This was courageous and potentially risky for the student in his down-power role. I could feel the energy in the room getting tense. The teacher responded quickly and skillfully. "Thank you for pointing this out, Sam. You're so right. I wasn't really listening to you. I was twisting what you said to make a point I wanted to make." I'm so sorry. I believe I did the same thing earlier with Carmen's comment. I will correct this. Please let me know if it happens again and I have missed it." Not only did the issue resolve, but also the students felt more trust and respect for the teacher. She did several important things in that brief response. She was not defensive, she gave a short and vulnerable explanation, she took responsibility for changing her habit, and she apologized. It took all of two minutes.*

Although we usually focus, rightly, on the feelings and needs of the hurt person, I got interested in what happens for the apologizer when they apologize: "I got to let go of at least some of my guilt by taking responsibility for my offending behavior." "Surprisingly, the relationship got better!" "In finally facing up to the harm I'd caused, I learned something about myself and some habits that I didn't like. This was the first step toward changing them." "I learned that it's really okay to make mistakes. What isn't okay is not to apologize and learn from them."

Making a worthy apology is far more complex than a simple "I'm sorry." John Kador[cxvi] has written a whole book about the process of making an effective apology. He describes five dimensions[cxvii] that are involved in an effective apology. These are similar to the five aspects of resolving difficulties discussed in this chapter.

1. Recognition. Apology requires your recognition that what you did was wrong and harmful. The injured person needs to know that you understand your offense and that you are apologizing for the right thing: with no "ifs or buts." "I'm sorry I hurt you, (too vague) or, I'm sorry you were hurt," (no personal responsibility) are not sufficient. "I'm sorry I spoke to you in a disrespectful way" is better because it names specific behavior. It is more effective when both parties agree on the facts of what happened, but sometimes when there is disagreement, you need to give up your need for this aspect of closure. "Apology is basically giving up our struggle with history."[cxviii]

2. Responsibility. In this dimension you take full responsibility for your offense without being defensive, making excuses, offering long explanations, or blaming anyone else. "You misunderstood me. What I meant was. . . . *or* What's your part in this?" won't get you very far and might even make matters worse. Explanations tend to burden apologies and serve the needs of the apologizer more than the one who was wronged. However, there are times, as mentioned on page 170, when speaking of your intention is important and helpful.

3. Remorse. Here you use the words, "I'm sorry, or I apologize, or here's what I regret." It seems there isn't any substitute for these exact words accompanied by appropriate feeling. Begin with "I" to make it clear that this is a personal response from you.

4. Restitution. You need to make amends. You need to offer an appropriate action. Restitution should be aimed at a repair that goes one step beyond the actual harm done. "I was twenty minutes late for our appointment. I'm so sorry. I get it that you felt anxious and worried. I'd like to offer you the whole session today without charge." Your offer shows respect and a deep level of willingness to take responsibility for the repair. Sometimes, however, it can be okay to begin the repair conversation by asking what would be needed for repair.

5. Repetition. Here is where you say what you have learned, how you have changed and how things will be different in the future. This is your commitment to not repeat the offending action. For example, "I have learned that I have poor boundaries. I revealed confidential information about you, causing you a lot of pain. I will not do this again. I hope that over time you will be able to trust me again."

When an offense is small, simple and immediate is better. "I'm sorry." When the offense is great, take some time to think it through. Beware of habitually apologizing and habitually avoiding apologizing.

The other side of offering an apology is accepting one. On the receiving side you must discern whether the apology is genuine and also whether it feels satisfactory. Accepting is just accepting. It doesn't automatically include trusting or forgiving. Rebuilding trust happens over time. Forgiveness is a separate process. When the apology is genuine, it is important to say, "I accept your apology." The interaction needs to be complete and acknowledged.

Apology can move mountains. A half-hearted one can make things worse. A sincere and well-crafted apology can restore relationships. Right Use of Power teacher, Michael Moore has an easy-to-remember acronym: **CARE**. **C**ontent, **A**ffect, **R**esponsibility, **E**mpathy.

6. The Power of Forgiveness

In the largest context, forgiveness has the awesome power to stop the cycles of revenge and violence that drive egregious abuses of power. Luskin says, "By choosing to forgive, we stand in awe of the horrors that can happen to people in this world and we decide neither to participate in them nor to repay them. It's not a matter of whether or not we will have conflict; it's a matter of what we do with that conflict."

Forgiveness is often misunderstood. It does not require forgetting or condoning or even reconciling. Fred Luskin[cxix] defines forgiveness as "the ability to make peace with your own life by no longer arguing and objecting to the way it unfolds. It means that difficult things happen in life, and first you have to grieve them, then accept them, and finally move on. . . . Forgiveness means that unkindness stops with you. . . . This is not a one-time response. . . . It's about becoming a forgiving person." Vesala Simic[cxx] adds, "Forgiveness is a pro-social change in someone's experience after a transgression. When people choose to forgive, they change."

Forgiveness is the end-point of a process of coming to terms with enormous harm and with the reverberations of that harm. Forgiveness is ultimately liberating and life-restoring. Although it is about a relationship, forgiveness is for yourself. "Instead of letting the person who caused the harm, 'off the hook,' forgiveness is about taking the hooks of hurt, anger, and helplessness out of our aching hearts so we can grieve and heal and let go of destructive feelings," as Jack Lavino[cxxi] puts it.

Jack describes several stages of forgiveness that are best worked through with the support of a therapist or other professional. The first is to break the silence and tell the story to someone who is safe. Next, is to allow yourself to feel and grieve. The next stage is to take responsibility for your own reactions to pain. And the last stage is to accept the humanity of your abuser. By forgiving the unforgiveable, you, or your client gains freedom from responses of revenge, further suffering, martyrdom, rage, helplessness, and re-traumatizing. The energy that has held the pain and anger is released and you can move on. The deadly repeating cycle stops. "Forgiveness is not for sissies. It is the hero's journey."[cxxii]

The ethical consideration in working with forgiveness with clients is in understanding that getting to forgiveness is a long and deep engagement with Self that can't be pushed or forced. There is a moment when forgiveness feels possible and right. Pushing for it before there has been adequate grieving, expression of anger, and understanding of the beliefs, habits and addictions that have resulted from the wound, can have the unintended effect of increasing shame and anger and decreasing trust.

Story: Carla was angry with her father for being so selfish and crazy that he expected her from the time she was a small child and her parents divorced, to take care of him and make him happy. He frequently threatened to kill himself if she didn't do something for him. She was upset that as a child she had made it her life purpose to take care of her father. Sessions cycled through anger and grief. Her insight that in her adult relationships she was either a resentful caretaker or withdrawn and unavailable, gave her strong motivation to get out of this endless cycle of hatred. In one session I asked her to select something in the room to represent her Dad. She found a jar and placed it in the room at a distance that felt right. At first, she was so angry that she couldn't even look at the jar. We acknowledged this and let it be. The next session the jar was still there. But now she could look at it. "I am thinking to go and pick it up and hold it. But I can't do that." (Tears) "It's not ME. He's not me. His life is not mine. It belongs to HIM." In that moment he became a very wounded but separate human being, instead of her life purpose and her tormentor. NOW she could forgive him and take back her own life.

Excellent resources on Forgiveness are abundant.[cxxiii]

7. The Power of Self-Correction

In self-correcting you are communicating and demonstrating that you have learned or understood something new about yourself, your client, or a professional issue. One of my teachers, Barney Aldrich, a master carpenter said, *"The sign of a good carpenter is not one who never makes mistakes, but one who knows how to fix them."*[cxxiv] These words provide a nice reframe for true mastery. In self-correcting you are embracing growth and normalizing the truth that mistakes and misunderstandings are inevitable. Self-correcting, itself, is a compassionate process unhindered by shame or blame.

8. The Power of Relationship Repair

Asking what is needed for relationship repair is usually experienced with relief and interest. In fact, one of my students wept when I asked her what was needed for relationship repair. She said no one had ever, during a conflict, demonstrated such concern for the relationship. This question acknowledges your confidence that the relationship can be repaired and the value you place on the relationship. People yearn to be connected and valued. Personal experience with relationship repair instead of relationship loss is touching and restorative. Once the relationship is repaired, the increased trust opens opportunities to honestly and productively explore with clients' wounds, habits, and beliefs that may cause relationship difficulties.

In practicing Right Use of Power, appropriately used expressions of apology, sorrow, and regret point the way to conflict resolution and relationship repair; and they require staying connected in the relationship.

9. *The Power of Preparing to Repair*

"The single most important determinant of how well repair of a disconnect goes is the quality of preparation," says my Hakomi colleague, Rhonda Mattern.   She adds, "I've found that jumping into a repair conversation without personally untangling at least some of their emotions, hurts, values, needs, and requests makes good repair almost impossible or requires multiple additional conversations that people tend not to schedule, leaving the repair unfinished."   She recommends speaking with someone you trust as you prepare. Especially helpful questions to reflect on are on page 221-222 in the Grievances chapter. In addition to being emotionally centered and available, it is very important to have identified your emotions and needs and the specific behavior you observed in the other person(s) that gave rise to those emotions and needs. In your meeting make a specific request of the other person(s) that would make the repair feel complete.

10. *The Power of Bracketing the Past*

Sometimes there is so much accumulated negative emotion, judgments, distrust, and complicated history in a relationship or set of relationships that the wisest thing is to bracket the past and focus instead on how you want to relate. I have experienced people and groups spending enormous amounts of time trying to heal every past interaction and only getting bogged down and frustrated. It takes skill and wisdom to let the past go and concentrate on creating agreements about how to relate more satisfactorily in the future.

Using the power spiral as a guide
Here's a description of how to use the power spiral as a guide for resolving difficulties.

Information—Recognize a Difficulty
Notice that there's some kind of difficulty or conflict. Track for indicators in your client's affect or behavior and/or in your own felt sense. (Remember that indicators may be very subtle and may vanish quickly if they are not noticed.)

Awareness—Acknowledge, understand, validate, and empathize
Check in with your client. *"Something seems to be upsetting you. Tell me about your experience."* (Remember that acknowledging your client's feelings and experience doesn't necessarily mean that you agree or have the same feelings or experience.) Your client simply needs to be understood and their complaint or upset validated. Be authentically compassionate and empathic.

Clarify what happened. *"Let's see if we can clarify what happened. You felt hurt when I said _____. I want you to know that it wasn't my intention to hurt you, but I can see how you felt the way you did. Have I understood accurately?"* (Remember that genuine concern, interest, non-defensiveness, and a willingness to turn toward conflict are your best allies.)

Accountability—Stay Connected, Resolve, and Repair
A simple and powerful way to shift from reacting to re-connecting, is to shift your attitude to curiosity. Become genuinely curious about your client and the situation. Curiosity is an antidote to judgment and fear.

When the timing is right, offer a simple apology or regret. *"I'm so sorry that I hurt you."* Or, *"I apologize for being late."* Or, *"I regret that I didn't ask you about that."* An apology can be about their hurt or your behavior.

Sometimes more is needed. *"I see that something else is needed to fully resolve this situation. What could be a next step toward resolution?"*

Give the relationship some attention. *"What is needed for relationship repair?"*

Empowerment—Self-correct and let go
Assure your client about the future. *"In the future I will arrange my schedule with more time between appointments."* (A self-correction should be behavioral, rather than *"I'll try."*)

Resource yourself. Reflect on the situation on your own, and/or in supervision. Self-correct as needed. Let go. Sometimes, even given the most skillful and earnest attention, situations do not resolve and relationships are not repaired. Knowing when to persist and when to let go, appropriately protecting yourself, grieving, letting time pass, and bringing your learnings to other situations can help.

Returning to the East in the spiral—Check in and go deeper
Check in with your client about how it's been going since the event. Most often the result of this process will be resolution of the difficulty and a deepening of trust and connectedness. When this is the case, use this increased trust and collaboration and go deeper, as appropriate to your modality.   Your goal in working with difficulties is to increase the integrity, trust, safety, and collaboration in the relationship.

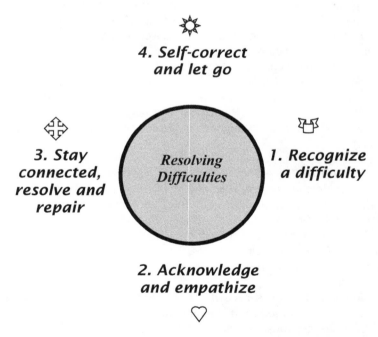

The following page charts another power spiral process for resolution.[cxxv]

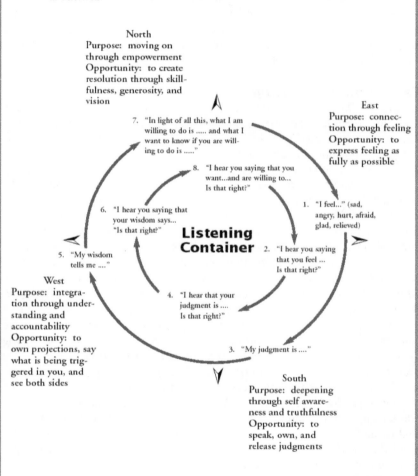

Using this process: Listener sits in the center in the listening container and receives the communications from each quadrant from the Talker, responding as described.

North
Purpose: moving on through empowerment
Opportunity: to create resolution through skillfulness, generosity, and vision

East
Purpose: connection through feeling
Opportunity: to express feeling as fully as possible

7. "In light of all this, what I am willing to do is ..... and what I want to know if you are willing to do is ....."

8. "I hear you saying that you want...and are willing to... Is that right?"

1. "I feel..." (sad, angry, hurt, afraid, glad, relieved)

6. "I hear you saying that your wisdom says... "Is that right?"

Listening Container

2. "I hear you saying that you feel ... Is that right?"

5. "My wisdom tells me ...."

4. "I hear that your judgment is .... Is that right?"

West
Purpose: integration through understanding and accountability
Opportunity: to own projections, say what is being triggered in you, and see both sides

3. "My judgment is ...."

South
Purpose: deepening through self awareness and truthfulness
Opportunity: to speak, own, and release judgments

Grievance Prevention

The experience of people serving on ethics committees,[cxxxvi] has been that many grievances were resolved simply by compassionate listening and acknowledgement of the claimant's experience by a committee member in a power position within the organization. Therapeutic relationships in which a conflict was well handled were experienced as more successful than therapeutic relationships that were smooth and conflict free. What is most important is not whether you make any mistakes or cause any harm, but how well you can resolve and repair.

Persisting and Letting Go

Story: During group process well into professional psychotherapy training, Gary, a Psychiatrist, began to speak. He was in quite a bit of distress and crying as he talked. "I'm not worthy of being a member of this group. I can't hide this anymore and you can tell me to leave if you want. But I need you to know that I abused my sisters when I was a teenager. I feel so bad about myself. I've asked them to forgive me, but they won't. It's so painful that they won't forgive me. And I can understand why they won't. Since they won't talk to me I had to do something, so I started doing what I can do instead of grieving over what I can't. I volunteer at the Rape Crisis Center. And I want you to know that I have broken the cycle of abuse in my family. I have not abused my daughters. What will you think of me now that you know this?" The room was silent while he wept for some minutes. A woman and a man both moved closer to him in silent support. When he was able to look up, someone in the group said, "I'm sorry that your sisters don't know your sorrow and who you've become, but I forgive you, and I'm proud of you and happy to be a friend and colleague." One by one, others nodded or repeated similar things as Gary looked around at each student. His tears now were those of relief, self-acceptance, and love.

Even after giving it your best, some conflicts don't resolve, and some relationships don't get repaired. When healing can't happen within the relationship, rather than let it fester in despair, anger, or helplessness, seek healing and/or resolution in other ways. It might be time to let it go. There is wisdom and courage in knowing when to persist and when to let go. Healing can happen in unexpected ways through:

- the passage of time
- experiencing things differently in another relationship
- grieving and forgiving
- using what you have learned to prevent similar harm
- the great mystery

Denial of Responsibility and/or Intentional Harm

There are a small percentage of practitioners who cause egregious harm to clients intentionally or not, through denial of their accountability, focusing blame away from themselves, and/or because they think they can get away with it. Their unethical behavior may be influenced by their own personal wounding, unresolved anger, low self-esteem, poor boundaries, personality disorder, projection, or shame.

Story: A grievance was brought against a bodyworker. The main evidence was a series of emails in which the bodyworker responded inappropriately and, in addition, refused several attempts at resolution initiated by the client. When this written record was brought to his attention, instead of responding with sorrow and a desire to repair and learn from this, the bodyworker began to shift the blame to the client, to the grievance committee and to the bodywork school he had attended. It seemed that the more sincerely the Grievance Committee attempted to respond, the greater the escalation of blame. The committee's goal was repair and re-education. However, the blame-shifting stopped only when the Committee set a boundary of no further communication. In this case the client felt heard and respected through the Grievance Process, but the bodyworker lost a chance to self-correct and continue with his practice.

For practitioners such as the one in this story, a grievance process was needed. Through the formal process, some caregivers can apologize and self-correct. Others will need to be removed from their professional practice. It is a professional responsibility to protect the public from harm and to protect practitioners from false accusations.

Unfair Accusations

There are of course, situations in which the caregiver is unfairly accused. In some of these, looking back in hindsight, it is clear that the problem could have been handled early on and/or that the escalation is actually a disguise for a deeper issue that is not being recognized or attended to. In other situations, it becomes clear, after genuine attempts to work on the issue and the relationship, that the client is responding from a character or addictive disorder, is not capable of resolving the issue, has another agenda, or is projecting and over-reacting. In this case, supervision, setting and holding clear boundaries, and keeping good records are the best protective measures.

Escalators

There are a small percentage of clients, students, parishioners, employees with whom conflict is not going to resolve. You may have contacted their feelings, been empathetic, apologized, asked them what they needed and all in all, spent an inordinate amount of time, energy and attention on them. Even when things seem to be resolved, the same issue arises again. I call these people Escalators. Why is there no settling, no stability, no resolution, no repair? Some are so wounded that they can't be in their social engagement nervous system. Some find negative connection better than no connection at all. Some seek revenge for hurts that may not even involve you. Some don't know how to connect, let alone repair, a broken relationship. Some have a strong need for control to offset their vulnerability. Some have a personality disorder that interferes. Some are just mean or vengeful.

What to do? You bear 150% responsibility for the health of the relationship. At the same time, it is not your job to be used or abused. The first thing is to recognize Escalator behavior early on. Look for characteristics: something seems resolved but isn't; they can't answer a question about what they would need to feel resolved or what they want is unrealistic or impossible; you don't feel connected; the energy keeps building instead of settling; their responses seem out of proportion or irrational; they seem to need an inordinate or unrealistic amount of your attention; they focus on extraneous details instead of the real issue.

What to do? Here's where you need to lean in to the strength aspect of your power. Be kind and respectful, yes. Feel your compassion for whatever is interfering with coming to resolution and repair. But begin, as soon as you suspect an Escalator, clarifying, setting, and maintaining good boundaries. Offering more and more and more time, attention, understanding and open-endedness when it is not leading to more clarity, trust, or ease is actually likely to support and even increase the escalation and intensity. Use your up-power role to set specific expectations about goals, behaviors, time frames and consequences. In the end setting firmer and firmer boundaries or even removing the escalator from a group may be letting go of small kindness in trade for greater kindness. Guidance from a supervisor or a consultant can be of help in staying centered and firm and deciding how to proceed.

I hear disturbing stories from kind and compassionate therapists and leaders who end up feeling frustrated, weary, and upset by the very people they are trying to treat with kindness alone. After spending some time with the leader of a spiritual center listening to her experience of being with a student who as an "escalator," I asked her if she had any suggestions to offer others. In her situation, after this leader had spent two years patiently addressing the escalation and trying to resolve the conflict, the student filed a grievance and consulted a lawyer. It all ended when the student was finally advised not to pursue this any further in a public way because what she was doing could legally be considered defamation of character. Here are her wise words. (She did add that these are not the things she necessarily did or did well, but are, in hindsight helpful ways to think about things and to respond.)

1. "Try to stay calm. It's so easy to get caught obsessing over the situation--the unfairness of it, the damage it is causing, the speculation about what went wrong, what was said, what was intended, and so on. You can get trapped in the spin of it and this is a great danger. Like the shame dungeon, getting caught in that way de-resources you and makes it impossible to think clearly and respond appropriately.

2. It becomes difficult to find your natural compassion for someone who seems bent on causing pain for you or those you care about. It might help to remember that the pain you are experiencing is a reflection of the pain and distress the person is desperately trying to offload. Although they may be gratified by seeing you in distress, it's very important not to provide that gratification, to be contained and hold firmly to keeping the focus on their process. Save your upset for your own therapist or supervisor or trusted consultant. If you don't have one, get one.

3. You will likely recognize that there is some seed of truth in what the other person is saying, for example, something they accurately observed, but most likely the interpretation or meanings they've given to it is far off the mark. Although you might clarify your intention or motive once or twice, don't get into repeated loops about "what you really meant," or "what you actually said." Once you've provided your explanation, simply say, "We've discussed this before, you've explained your perspective and I've explained my perspective, and there is really no point in going over it again. You do not seem satisfied, somehow, but there's no point in revisiting the same ground unless there is something new to add."

4. The core accusation seems to be your failure of perfect care. Because we are in care-giving professions or callings, this charge is especially painful. We can accept our mistakes of technique, skill, or method, but we are devastated by the reflection that we do not live up to our deep intentions and aspirations. And in the situation, you may actually feel a loss of compassion and care for the person who is causing you so

much distress, seemingly through malice. This is a sign of how grave the situation really is, as a threat to your own sense of who you are. Don't worry, you are not actually uncaring or uncompassionate. You do not need to find another profession, as you may feel desperately inclined to do. This is not a person who has deeply seen through you and discovered your deepest lack, hidden to the rest of the world; it is a person who has tapped into that particular fear you carry. You lack nothing that you need to respond wisely and compassionately in any situation. But you are human. You have limits.

5. The situation is likely to escalate beyond what you could possibly predict. Be prepared for surprises: the person writes a letter to your professional board or association condemning you and seeking your punishment or public disgrace. Or the person invades your personal life, contacting friends or relatives to hear the accusations. The person may say that this information is "confidential," and so you may not know right away that the damage is happening. This is particularly painful and requires a lot of fortitude, as you patiently, clearly, and kindly respond to the concerns expressed by others. Or the person may post the accusations and criticisms online. Stop. Don't attempt to get into a public, online "correction" or battle. Remember that any public figure gets this kind of thing daily, so you might as well feel famous.

6. Hold a firm line. Let the person know that if they persist, they are crossing the line into legal sanctions, for example harassment and defamation. This is of course the "nuclear option." Except in very particular circumstances, you would not press a lawsuit against the person, but they need to know that the behavior they are engaging in is actually proscribed by law.

7. Stay connected to sources of nourishment and care for yourself. Remember that this kind of behavior is the exception, statistically a very tiny percentage of the people you deal with, and of people in the world. Don't allow that tiny percentage to contaminate your other relationships, destroy your faith in what you are doing, or deter you on your path."

Summary: Some Principles for Conflict Resolution

- What people with complaints need most is empathy—a sincere demonstration of understanding and validating their experience. Empathy is most simply conveyed in words such as . . . ."When I _____, it makes you feel _____."

- Acquiring a positive and confident relationship with conflict begins with disassociating trauma from conflict. Conflict does not automatically produce trauma and relationship loss.[cxxvii]

- Remember that trauma and shame jeopardize people's ability to be in relationship, be resourced, and reality check. They will then be less capable or unable to resolve things in a rational, reasonable, and relational way.

- Seek to understand the unmet needs of each party. Identifying specific unmet needs reveals the opposite—creative ways for everyone's needs to be met.[cxxviii]

- Be personal. Talk about your experience and invite others to do the same.

- Link complaints with requests for change and ask for specific suggestions.

- Hold your seat at the same time you soften with compassion.

- Remember and appreciate your resilience and those of others.

- Be led by curiosity.

- Everyone has some piece of the truth. Look for ways to recognize and appreciate this truth and the good intentions behind it.

- Acknowledge and appreciate good intentions, and understand that impact may be different than intention.

- Endeavor to understand your own history, motivations, habits, and beliefs around power.

- Develop your capacity to witness. Witnessing is a powerful position. Take a balcony view.[cxxix]

- Have faith in the possibility of relationship repair.

- Ask for feedback about your impact.

- Focus on feelings, needs, and requests.

- Be patient and let go of being attached to a particular outcome. Resolution may happen in a form or timing that might surprise you.

- Pay attention to when to persist and when to let go.

- Distinguish between unintentional and intentional harm and be willing and courageous about using your power to take a firm and direct stand when this is needed.

> *"Madame, do I not destroy my enemies, when I turn them into friends?"*   —*Abraham Lincoln*[cxxx]

> *"If you want to make peace, you don't talk to your friends, you talk to your enemies."*   —*Moshe Dayan*[cxxxi]

Additional great resources

Seven specific resources for further study of conflict resolution

Appreciative Inquiry[cxxxii]

Tom Osborn and others work with corporations through what they call Appreciative Inquiry. Instead of the usual problem-solving process of identifying all the problems and all their awful results, probing into the causes, analyzing possible solutions, and then enacting remedies, Osborn begins by asking the people he meets to name all the things that are working in the organization. He then helps them envision what might be, dialogue about what should be, and innovate what will be. This, he says, *"creates an environment in which the generative and creative forces in the organization provide the energy to move forward. Rather than denying problems, it redefines them."* He adds that *"the forward motion of moving toward an image rather than the backward look at what is wrong.... enables organizations to be agile and.... embrace the rapid change that is the water in which we swim. . . .Positive image creates positive action, which produces positive outcomes."*

Marshall Rosenberg: Non-Violent Communication

Concerned about the prevalence, destructiveness, and ineffectiveness of violence as a method for handling conflict, both locally and internationally, Marshall Rosenberg developed a philosophy and tool for successful conflict management called Nonviolent Communication (NVC). In an article from the magazine *"Shift,"*[cxxxiii] Rosenberg says he was motivated to find out *"what happens to disconnect us from our compassionate nature, and what allows some people to stay connected to their compassionate nature under even the most trying circumstances." From this inquiry, he decided that violence did not arise from pathology, as he had been taught, but from the ways in which we communicate."*

Rosenberg's Nonviolent Communication has four steps:

1. *observing what is happening in a given situation;*
2. *identifying what one is feeling;*
3. *identifying what one is needing;*
4. *then making a request for what one would like to see occur.*

This inspiring story is from an interview. [cxxxiv]

Marshall Rosenberg: "When you get people to talk about what they want from each other, instead of what's wrong with the other, there's a possibility for reconciliation to begin."

IM: Could you give us a concrete example from the international work that you've done in conflict resolution?

Marshall Rosenberg: "About eight years ago, I was mediating between a Muslim tribe and a Christian tribe in northern Nigeria. In their conflict, a quarter of the population had been killed. At that time, they were fighting about how many places in the marketplace each side would have to display their products. I started the reconciliation process with them by saying that I was confident that if we could hear each other's needs, we could find a way to get everybody's needs met. Inviting whoever wanted to start, I asked: "What needs of yours are not getting met?" The chief from the Christian tribe screamed, "You people are murderers!" Notice that when I asked him what needs weren't getting met, his response was to tell me what was wrong with the other side. This provoked a counter judgment. Somebody on the Muslim side screamed back, "You've been trying to dominate us! We're not going to tolerate it anymore!"

Because our training is based on the assumption that all violent language is a tragic expression of unmet needs, when the chiefs finished screaming, my job was to translate the enemy image of "murderer" into language describing the needs of the person who screamed. I said, "Chief, are you saying that your need for safety is not being met and you want some agreement that no matter what the conflict, that it be resolved some way other than violence?" He looked shocked for a moment because this is different from how people are trained to think. Then he said, "That's exactly right."

But getting the chief to acknowledge his need wasn't enough. I had to get the Muslim side to see through their enemy image. I said, "Would somebody on the other side please tell me what you heard the chief say his needs were?"

A gentleman from the Muslim tribe screamed back, "Then why did you kill my son?" In fact, there were several others in the Muslim tribe who knew that someone present had killed one of their children. So, there were a lot of feelings. The Muslim tribe had to put down their rage long enough to hear the needs of the Christian tribe. And that wasn't easy. I had to give them some empathy before they could do that. But finally, I got them to hear just one simple thing, that the Christian tribe had said they had a need for safety.

It took me about an hour and a half to get both sides to release the enemy image long enough to hear a need of the other side. At that point, one of the chiefs came up and said to me, "If we know how to communicate this way, we don't have to kill each other!"

Rosenberg explains that his "trainings are based on an assumption that when we are clear and connected to ourselves, there's nothing that we like better than to contribute to one another's well-being. But there are a number of things that can happen to disconnect us from that. So, for me, reconciliation is connecting people again so they enjoy contributing to each other's well-being rather than contributing to each other's suffering. By 'connecting' I mean clearly seeing what's alive in one another, with no enemy images."

IM: "Hatred is so addictive. It often seems that feelings like empathy and understanding don't have a chance."

Rosenberg: "No matter what pain has gone on, if we connect people in a human way, their nature is to reconcile and to understand each other's needs. What's more addictive than hatred is compassion."

William Ury: "The Third Side: Why We Fight and How We Can Stop." [cxxxv];also," Difficult Conversations," by Stone, Patton, Heen

International negotiator, Bill Ury, teaches people to take the Third Side as a way of looking at conflicts not just from one side or the other, but from the larger perspective of the surrounding community. This Third Side has three components (called balconies): the emotional, the rational, and the creative. Going to the Third Side is a place to stop, look inside, and listen and hold a larger container where a creative and compassionate alchemy can result in a solution that respects the needs of all sides. From the Third Side perspective it becomes easier to differentiate between positions (which can become rigid) and interests (which open the door to creative win/win resolutions). For Ury, the purpose is not to reach an agreement, but to meet underlying needs. The goal is not to make all conflict disappear, but to transform conflict from destructive to constructive.

Shauna Ries and Susan Harter: In Justice, in Accord[cxxxvi]

Shauna Ries and Genna Murphy are co-founders of an organization called *Mediators without Borders* and have developed an extensive and internationally effective mediation process and training program. As they describe it in the forward, they "articulate a method. . . . that honors the full capacities of each individual disputant, including their emotions as well as their thoughts, their feelings and their bottom-lines. . . . The *inAccord* model has as its core the concept that individuals can find the shared means to create the interpersonal justice that they desire."

International Four Point Tool for Conflict Resolution[cxxxvii]

(Before any negotiation, each country is required to complete a four-point assessment. This includes negotiations around deep conflicts in world trouble spots.)

1) *What am I noticing, how do I see, what is my perspective on this issue?*

2) *How do I feel about what I see or am noticing? How do I feel about this issue?*

3) *What do I want or need or desire surrounding this issue?*

4) *What am I willing to do or not willing to do about this issue*

Navajo Elders prescription for conflict resolution[cxxxviii]

1) *Gratitude*

2) *What's working*

3) *What's not working?*

4) *Present at least 3 creative solutions.*

(You need at least 10 to show that you've stretched beyond your position.)

Conflict Resolution Network

From "Fighting Fair: A Conflict Resolution Guide"

1. *Do I want to resolve the conflict?*
   Be willing to fix the problem.

2. *Can I see the whole picture, not just my own point of view?*
   Broaden your outlook.

3. *What are the needs and anxieties of everyone involved?*
   Write them down.

4. *How can we make this fair?*
   Think up as many solutions as you can. Pick the one that gives everyone what they want.

5. *Can we work it out together?*
   Treat each other as equals.

6. *What am I feeling?*
   Am I too emotional? Could I get more facts, take time out to calm down, tell them how I feel?

7. *What do I want to change?*
   Be clear. Attack the problem, not the person.

8. *What opportunity can this bring?*

Work on the positives, not the negatives.
9.   *What is it like to be in their shoes?*
     Do they know I understand them?

> *"Maturity is the ability to find the similarities in the apparently different and the differences in the apparently similar. The goal is to differentiate and then integrate these differences."*
> —*Yvonne Agazarian*[cxxxix]

> *"God grant me the Serenity to accept the things I cannot change, the Courage to change the things I can; Wisdom to know the difference, and Strength to try to change what should be changed even when the change cannot be immediately effected."*
> —*(addition from Robbins Barstow*[cxl]*)*

> *"He drew a circle that shut me out—*
> *Heretic, rebel a thing to flout,*
> *But love and I had the wit to win:*
> *We drew a circle that took him in."*   —*Edwin Markham*[cxli]

> *"There is ninety percent agreement cross-culturally about the causation of conflict: People who do not say what they mean. People who do not do what they say."*   —*Angeles Arrien*[cxlii]

Self-study

1) Skillfulness in resolving and repairing difficulties comes with practice. For self-study, notice how you feel about conflict. Is it connected with trauma for you? Identify your habitual ways of avoiding conflict. Create in your mind a "new story" about how you want to respond to and use conflict.

2) Reflect on several situations in which a difficulty did NOT get resolved well. What kinds of impairment may have contributed to the lack of success? (I.e. see on page 9 a list of interferences with right use of power.) If you could do it over, what would you do differently to get a more successful outcome?

3) Now reflect on a situation in your current life that remains unresolved. What would you need, in yourself, and from the other for this to resolve and repair?   Now, imagine these things that you need in yourself and from the other actually having happened. What does this feel like?   Perhaps   reflecting on this gives you an idea of something you can do in yourself or something specific you could ask for.

4) Here are several examples of <u>ineffective</u> apologies.   Notice what doesn't work about each one.
> *"I'm sorry you were hurt."*
> *"Well, nobody's perfect."*
> *"So, sorry. Now let's move on."*
> *"You misunderstood me. What I meant was. . . ."*
> *"You made that up."*
> *"I'm sorry I hurt you."*
> *"What's your part in this?"*
> *"I was under a lot of stress and feeling badly at the time."*
> *"I should have apologized earlier."*
> *"There's really nothing for me to apologize about."*
> *"We were both wrong."*
> *"I was maybe a little bit unskillful."*
> *"I didn't help you handle the situation better."*
> *"There was a relationship change. You just didn't adjust. Sorry."*
> *"I did the best I could. I'm sorry it wasn't good enough for you."*

Grievance Processes

Sentences like, "I'm going to file an ethical grievance about you" or "I'm going to take you to court over this," can be used as an appropriate response to injustice or harm, as a threat to intimidate or control, or as a means to bring serious attention to a situation. Let's de-mystify what actually happens when a complaint is made.

Egregious violence, racism, and sexual abuse aside, most people, when they feel wounded or mistreated, want any or all of the following surprisingly simple things:

- *Acknowledgment and understanding of impact*
- *Clarification of intention*
- *Simple apology*
- *Self-correction or new understanding*
- *Relationship Repair or conscious closure*

When difficulties are not noticed or attended to within the relationship, the situation can escalate surprisingly quickly to a grievance or lawsuit. If resolution is not acquired at one level, the complaint is likely to escalate to the next level of severity. The following progression describes the escalation process.

6. Legal action
5. Grievance filed with a professional organization, state Grievance Board or a legal action
4. Mediated resolution
3. Conversation with a third-party present
2. Personal conversation at a later time
1. Simplest, most satisfying, and effective is personal conversation in the moment.

Complaints at the formal grievance or lawsuit level are lengthy, expensive, and stressful. Results tend to be less satisfactory than personal or mediated resolution. In addition, as a conflict escalates, there is an increasing likelihood of traumatic responses from both or either sides.

When asked to notice their immediate response to hearing, "An ethical grievance has been filed against you," practitioners said, "fear, shame, horror, bracing, shutting down, surprise, tears, threat, curiosity, self-righteousness, distress, fear of loss of livelihood, anger..." Being accused is an intense experience and many self-protective defenses arise. Here are some actual examples of counter-productive defensive responses to receiving a grievance letter: *"I shouldn't be bound by the guidelines at all because what I'm doing is not really therapy." "I can't afford supervision and no supervisor would understand what I do anyway." "I don't want to enroll in a grievance process that is based in a system I don't believe in." "If they really understood the situation, they wouldn't feel I had done anything wrong." "The problem isn't with my boundaries, it is that I'm simply too generous and people take advantage of me."*

Janet Thomas has done research on the impact on psychologists of receiving a licensing board complaint. She found that "psychologists become vulnerable to cognitive, emotional, and behavioral responses that may compromise their clinical work as well as their ability to defend themselves."[cxliii] They also are impaired in their ability to resolve the conflict. These responses include shame, cognitive fallacies that justify unethical behavior, depression, denial or over-confidence, anxiety, impaired objectivity, counter-transference, and self-defeating behaviors. It is valuable to know what these normal, although harmful, reactions can be because even with our best intentions and our most skillful attention, we are misunderstood, use poor judgment, or make mistakes, and can be grieved.

To summarize, ethical grievances or legal actions result when there has been significant harm caused by unethical behavior or when personal or mediated attempts at resolution have not been successful. Formal grievance and legal processes are intense and generally painful for both parties. Escalated fear, anger, defenses, distortions, and denial can impede and lengthen the process to months or even years.

Understandably, we don't want to go through a grievance process at all. Grievance processes are difficult situations and don't provide completion or the kind of satisfaction that comes through mediation or resolution within the relationship.

Grievance processes and litigation are designed to...
- *protect clients from harm*
- *protect practitioners from false accusations*
- *redress or repair harm to clients*
- *appropriately restrict further practice and/or re-educate practitioners*

Ethical Grievance Procedures
There are three basic kinds of ethical grievance procedures.

1) Grievance handled by state level Grievance Board.
This is a formal procedure in which a case is "heard" by members of an Ethics Board. Determinations are made about fault and appropriate actions are taken and administered. Cases accepted for review by State Grievance Boards tend to involve complex and thorough investigations.

2) Grievance handled by the Ethics Committee of a professional organization.
Because of the expense and expertise required to conduct a formal investigation, these in-house grievance procedures instead, are designed to facilitate all parties in hearing each other and in being heard by an unbiased committee within the organization.

3) Ethics complaint handled through litigation.
In this process, the claimant initiates legal action either as a first choice, or because they have tried other avenues without satisfaction. The legal system focuses on determining the one party as guilty and awarding punishment and/or financial redress.

Two Approaches for Handling Grievances
There are two quite different approaches to addressing grievances.

The traditional one is the legal system or jurisprudence. One of my students described his experience of formal grievance process as an "arm of the law." The focus of jurisprudence is on the ethic of justice. The process of determining who's right and who's wrong often includes adversarial exchanges and is a lengthy and expensive process. This focus can have the unintended result of escalating blame, self-righteousness, and lack of truthfulness since one party will be acquitted or judged guilty and punished. In this setting, taking responsibility for harm or making an apology can be used against the therapist. Most states require mental health professionals to take a jurisprudence class in which they are taught how to protect themselves from legal action by keeping the laws and proper documentation.

A second approach could be called relationship-prudence. Right use of power ethics uses relationship-prudence as a foundation. In this approach the focus is on the ethic of care. According to Carol Gilligan, [cxliv] "an ethic of justice proceeds from the premise of equality—that all should be treated the same," while "an ethic of care rests on the premise of non-violence— that no one should be harmed." Relationship-prudence focuses on pro-active resolution of conflict through

- Tracking for, and attending to difficulties within the relationship before they escalate
- Using conflict (instead of avoiding and fearing it) to build trust by clarifying and repairing relationships
- Examining mistakes and self-correcting for the future
- Practicing pro-active ethical decision-making

Ethics Committees--Relationship-Prudence

Small organizations[cxlv] for helping professionals in particular modalities, do not have the financial or personnel resources to conduct formal investigations of complaints in the way that state level grievance boards and lawyers can. These organizations can empower ethics committees to support resolution through facilitating honest communication, apology and reparative resolution. They can also assign appropriate re-education activities. Their goal is to maintain the ethical integrity of the organization by providing a process for responding to ethical complaints and resolving conflicts. They hold their practitioners accountable and provide education, guidance, advice and counsel so that unethical behaviors are not repeated.[cxlvi] Because they are relationship-prudent and resolution-focused, these organizations conduct interviews instead of investigations and reviews instead of formal processes. Here's an example of a review process used by a number of small organizations.

Review Process: Interview Stage

After being contacted by the claimant, two members of the ethics committee set up a separate phone call or in-person meeting with each party. The review is held in confidentiality. The interviewers conduct the interviews with compassionate questions aimed at empathizing, clarifying, and understanding what happened from both parties. For the claimant (the person bringing the complaint) there are questions such as: *What happened? Have you made any attempts to resolve this? What would you like to see happen here? Do you have any fears about what could happen?* For the respondent (the person being complained about) there are questions such as: *What happened? Have you made any attempts to resolve this? What would you like to see happen here? Do you have any fears about what might happen? How is it for you to hear this complaint? Is there anything you are sorry about? "What are you learning from this? If a similar situation came up again, would you respond differently and if so, how?*

The up-power party (the respondent) is considered to be 150% responsible for the health of the relationship and so it is acknowledged that the primary focus of the review process is on satisfactory resolution for the down-power party (the claimant). For the up-power party the focus is on clarification, truth, self-reflection, repair and personal learning. (There are situations in which both parties have equal role power--colleagues, for example, and are then equally responsible.)

Resolution Stage--Four Choices

Following the initial interviews with each party, the ethics committee members working with the case have several choices to make. They can take no action. They can suggest that further attempts be made to resolve the matter before bringing the situation back to the ethics committee. They can take the case forward as an ethical review. Or, if they decide the complaint is a dispute rather than an ethical violation, they can move forward with a conflict resolution process.

1) No Action

The committee members may take no action if they feel that everything that can be done to resolve things has been done and that further action by the committee will be unlikely to reach a more complete solution. They may also choose no action if the issue is deemed not appropriate for the ethics committee.

2) Suggest Other Avenues

The ethics committee may feel that the parties could be successful by doing more processing on their own or with the assistance of a colleague. After more attempts the parties would report resolution or return the matter to the committee. Depending on the situation, both disputants or an up-power disputant might be offered some questions to consider separately or together to facilitate their self-reflection and growth through working with the conflict. Here are a few sample questions. *Clarify what you already know about the issue. What do you want to happen? Why does this matter to you? What are you making up about the other person? What do you think you would need in yourself and from the other(s) for this to resolve?*

What are you afraid will happen? What part of this situation are you willing to acknowledge that you contribute to? Is there anything connected to your past here? If you let go of pride, being right, or your position, would it make a difference? What is the meaning or purpose of this issue or situation in your life? If you had a do-over, what would you do differently? What is your attachment to this situation? What do you think is at the core? What are you learning? What changes will you make so that this won't happen again?[cxlvii]

3) Ethical Review

If the complaint is determined to be a possible ethical violation, the review team will conduct additional interviews to get truth and clarity about the possible violation. They will then determine and apply appropriate responses aimed at re-education, such as requiring the practitioner to take a specific ethics course, get a certain amount of extra supervision, make a sincere apology, or write a paper describing his or her learnings. The purpose of these requirements would be to prevent future breaches.

4) Conflict Resolution

To assist in conflict resolution, the members of the ethics committee can facilitate communication between the two parties by listening from an objective and compassionate perspective and offering options and guidance. They can also serve as intermediaries for the clear transfer of information between the two parties. Or they can recommend a mediation process with trained mediators. Sometimes what is most needed by the claimant and/or respondent is guidance in discerning when and how to let go even when the situation was not successfully resolved.

There are several other factors to note. One is that sometimes the claimant simply needs to be compassionately acknowledged, listened to, and empathized with by the ethics committee. Receiving these things, the claimant decides that this is all that was needed and chooses to let it go. Another factor is that by correctly identifying a complaint as a dispute rather than an ethical grievance allows the ethics committee to simply offer guidance and support in resolving the situation. Without this option, people often feel that they need to find or escalate to an ethical breach in order to get help.

These alternative and relationship-prudent in-house processes can often prevent the filing of state level grievances and legal actions.

State Level Grievance Process

State Grievance Boards tend to use a combination of jurisprudence and relationship-prudence by basing their considerations on justice, remediation and re-education. Restorative Justice programs, for example, use the following three questions: *Who was harmed? Who is responsible? How can this harm be repaired?*

Some states have a mandatory informed consent document that each client must sign. It is designed to educate clients about what behaviors are unethical and to empower the client to do something about such behavior outside the client/therapist relationship if needed.

Generally, the claimant contacts the state or professional organization's grievance board or ethics committee and follows a set of procedures. These include writing a formal letter describing the grievance. The letter is then reviewed by the board and accepted or dismissed. When the complaint is accepted for further review, a copy of the complaint is sent to the Respondent (the person being grieved) for their written response.

The State Grievance Board has a number of possibilities for Disciplinary Sanctions. [cxlviii]

1) ***Letter of Admonition:*** This is the lowest level of disciplinary action that a board can impose. It consists of a written advisement to the psychotherapist that the Board has determined that the conduct complained of was an ethical violation.

2) ***Probation***: The practitioner is allowed to keep her/his license and continue practice under specific terms and conditions.

3) ***Suspension:*** This is a temporary loss of licensure privileges.

4) ***Revocation***: A permanent loss of licensure privileges.

5) ***Stipulated injunction***: An agreement between the Board and practitioner specifying the terms and/or conditions under which he/she may continue practice.

6) ***Injunction***: Terms and/or conditions under which the practitioner may practice are imposed, but there is no pre-agreement between the Board and the practitioner.

7) ***Cease and Desist***: An order for an immediate termination of practice.

Disciplinary actions numbers 2, 5, and 6 are the ones focused on re-education and self-correction on the part of the respondent. Requirements include taking specific and appropriate courses, supervision with written reports from the supervisor, and limitations on types of clients the therapist is permitted to work with.

Who Minds the Minders?[cxlix] What happens when Grievance Boards misuse their power? Right Use of Power teacher, Steve Vinay Gunther researched and published an excellent article that discusses issues and situations in which Grievance Boards have themselves acted unethically in their procedures and disciplinary actions. Here's the link: http://depth.net.au/Resources/Who_Minds_the_Minders.pdf

When Mediation is not Appropriate

Even when using relationship-prudence as a first and preferred method of resolving difficulties, there are situations in which a formal grievance procedure or legal action are necessary and appropriate. Here are some of these situations:

- practitioner is willfully and consistently violating ethical code
- practitioner is being falsely accused
- there has been sexual intimacy or abuse
- client or practitioner is too traumatized to have personal contact
- efforts at personal or mediated resolution have not been successful
- clear or suspected racism or discrimination

False Accusations

When a practitioner is falsely or unfairly accused, any of the following may be going on;

- The specific problem (or a build-up of smaller issues) was not resolved within the relationship.
- The escalation is a disguise for a deeper issue that has not been resolved and/or recognized.
- The client is responding from a character or addictive disorder.
- The client has created a "set-up" in order to benefit from a lawsuit.
- The client is not capable of resolving the issue or of letting go.
- The client has another agenda.
- The client is projecting or over-reacting.
- The client may have received bad advice.
- The practitioner is in denial about the actual harm they have caused.

If you feel you have been falsely accused, your best protective measures are good supervision, setting and holding clear boundaries, and keeping good records.

Risk Management

Professional ethics courses and continuing education programs in many professions, in addition to mental health practitioners, now include a topic called "risk management." Certainly it is wise to be ethically well-educated and to know strategies for reducing the risk of causing harm, however, many of these risk management courses create a culture of fear, over-cautiousness and even paranoia. "Risk management is a term referring to the avoidance of certain practices and interventions by therapists--not because they are clinically ill-advised, unethical, harmful, or wrong, but because they may appear so to judges, juries, licensing boards, or ethics committees."[cl] In these courses, therapists are told NEVER to touch a client, NEVER to accept a gift, NEVER to conduct a session outside the office, NEVER to self-disclose. These are behaviors that are sometimes therapeutically beneficial to clients. In fact, not doing so could even be harmful to the client and the relationship. Ethics is, after all, doing what is in the best interest of our clients or students. Risk management courses are often created by insurance companies in an attempt to reduce the cost of malpractice suits. Strict following of the prescribed risk management strategies can turn practitioners into over-cautious, fearful, defensive people who are focused on taking care of themselves at the expense of their clients' best care. As Ofer Zur poignantly says, the risk-management approach "tends to replace what the therapist can offer of warmth, soul, spontaneity, and human connection with a prissy, unattractive defensiveness."[cli]

Summary

The many forms of grievance procedures are designed and intended to serve the important purpose of protection and prevention of harm to both client and practitioner. Attending to difficulties within the helping relationship can, in many if not most cases, prevent difficulties from escalating to formal grievances.

Ideally, for a grievance process to serve well, there are four main things that are needed by each party.

The ethics committee needs:
Resolution
Education
Appropriate consequences
Confidence in learning (that the offense won't be repeated)

The Claimant needs:
Resolution
Repair
To be heard and empowered
To feel that he/she has contributed to learning

The Respondent needs:
An advocate
Appropriate consequences
A re-entry path
Confidentiality

"Without intervention, we often hold onto wounds with great force and conviction. With the right intervention, these feelings can just relax, like a fist releasing tension."   Richard John Kinane, ethics committee member

Self-Study: Reflection

Take a minute to think about this. If an ethical grievance were filed against you, what might it be about? What kind of pro-activity on your part could prevent such a situation? What kinds of action could resolve the problem and repair the relationship if it did happen?

Making Referrals & Handling Completions

"Providing services outside area of competence" is the second most frequently filed grievance, and "failure to terminate" and "failure to refer" are in the top 10 most frequent complaints. [clii] It is clear that skill and sensitivity are needed because of the power differential to prevent harm and promote well-being when ending your relationship with clients. This is true in the case of referrals to another practitioner when your service is no longer needed.

Practically, this involves:

- Knowing your area of competence and level of expertise
- Defining and limiting what you're doing, both for yourself and for your clients.
- Accurately assessing the effectiveness of your work and knowing when the process is complete
- Keeping a list of other practitioners as referral sources

Sensitively and clearly referring or completing

Examples: • *"We are nearing completion of our therapy. Let's take a look your original goals and see where you are now. I am getting a sense that you don't need to come anymore."*

• *"I'm feeling that what I have to offer isn't what you need right now for your healing. I'd like to recommend that you make an appointment with..."*

• *"I'll be going on vacation in three months. I'll be traveling for two months. While I'm gone my back-up therapist will be available to you. When I return, you may wish to stay with him or return to seeing me."*

• *"I notice a lot of intense feelings and memories are arising when you have your massages. I think it would be really helpful for you to see a psychotherapist for processing and additional support."*

Often completing or referring is that simple and direct. However, the impact of the power differential on clients creates an increase in their vulnerability to rejection and criticism. Clients both need and want you to like them and be impressed by their progress. They want and need to be valued and respected.

From their increased vulnerability, any of the above kind, rational, and direct sentences can be misunderstood as rejection, disapproval, or abandonment. Termination that is not mutual or only partially mutual can cause great pain that can resurface even months after the actual termination. The therapy relationship is vulnerable and intimate. Clients may be working on issues of attachment and self-esteem that may get triggered by termination that is not of their choosing. Even professional reasons like changing job, going on sabbatical, being out of your area of expertise, or sexual attraction, don't matter when clients interpret the termination as rejection. Tracking for indicators from your client that they may have felt rejected or criticized is can help you take these feelings seriously and address them even though responses may not seem reasonable to you.

Allowing time for completion

In the Hakomi Method of Body Centered Psychotherapy, there is a chart describing the process of a psychotherapy session called the Four Quadrant Chart.[cliii] (This chart could be applied to most sessions with helping professionals.) In the first quadrant, your aim is to establish a healing relationship, attend to safety issues, and get clear about what the goal for the session is. In the second and third quadrants, your work is to set up and engage in a process that will lead toward accomplishing your goal. The task in the fourth quadrant is to acknowledge what occurred; integrate, complete, set up the next session, and make sure your client is ready to go back out into the world.

The quadrants are symbolically set at 15-minute intervals whereas in reality each quadrant takes its own organic and/or managed time period. In supervising psychotherapy students, I have found that the quadrant that consistently gets under-attended is the fourth quadrant—completing. Integrating and completing are an essential part of the process of healing and should not be undervalued. When you plan adequate time for completing, there will be space and time to track and attend to difficulties, misunderstandings, or feelings of rejection or disapproval.

Stories

Here are several stories from practitioners of skillful uses of power in situations in which referring or completing is challenging and complex.

• *"I found myself developing a sexual attraction to my client. This was unusual. I tried to take back the projection, but the therapeutic relationship began feeling odd and my client wasn't getting my best healing work. I decided to just tell him that it didn't seem like the right client/therapist match and that I felt he wasn't getting the quality of attention he deserved from me. I listened to his disappointment and also was surprised that he had felt something wasn't quite working too. I talked with him in detail about possible other therapists and I'm glad to say he did make a good connection with another."*

• *"I'm not sure how this happened, but I became unsure whether my client needed something beyond my level of expertise, or whether I was competent but just lacking in self-confidence. I mentioned my concern to my client and she didn't have any concern at all, but I knew that she would likely, because of the power differential, want to stay with me, someone she was already attached to, rather than feel like she was "too much." So I didn't altogether trust her response. I spoke with my supervisor and we decided that I would continue, while being watchful for new indicators. My confidence improved as I discovered I could handle these issues well enough."*

• *"My massage client began getting very triggered and having terrible traumatic memories just through massage. I did the best I could to help her ground herself and not re-traumatize, but it was becoming a frequent event. I told her I thought she needed some psychotherapy to deal with these memories, but she didn't want to even consider it. I then had to tell her that I couldn't continue with massage until she was doing some kind of work with the trauma, because I felt the triggering was becoming harmful to her. She felt rejected and upset, but, to my surprise, called me a few weeks later for a referral. I guess I did a good job of keeping the relationship open because she then called to thank me for "making" her work on these issues."*

• *"My relationship with a client got very enmeshed and I knew it didn't feel right to continue. I didn't want to make things even worse and so when she emailed me wondering if this was still working for me, I emailed her back, relieved, and said terminated with her. I was so surprised months later when I got a call from the Grievance Review Committee that this client had made a complaint about abandonment. This was so painful, but I actually learned a lot. I understood that in asking whether this was still working for me, she was asking for reassurance. I also learned that accepting what I thought was her decision to terminate by email was in fact an insensitive and rejecting thing. What she wanted from the complaint was an apology in which I took responsibility for my hurtful actions. Once I stopped being defensive and saw what my impact had been, I apologized, genuinely. This was what she needed. I am much wiser as a result.*

•*"I discovered how important it is for me to feel that my clients are getting their money's worth and so I keep processing up until the very last minute. One client would consistently tell me that she didn't remember the last session. It seemed that she needed time to be set aside for integrating at the end. She wasn't the only one who needed that completion time. I did too."*

• *"I was going on a 6-week vacation and one of my clients was very dependent on me. He wanted to just wait until I got back, but I felt strongly that he needed weekly sessions. After much processing, I suggested that he call my back-up therapist while he was in my office to set up a specific appointment. He did, and he went to the appointment."*

• *"This was strange. My client felt that he was getting so much help from working with me, but my perception was that he was quite attached to me and the safety of our relationship and didn't understand what results my bodywork should have. I needed to tell him that the work just wasn't getting the improvements in mobility that should be expected. I then recommended another modality. This was a hard one, because I really needed clients, and he was satisfied. But I wanted to be in integrity."*

Well-being

A helping relationship is a complex one. We may become so focused on problems and suffering that we lose sight of the qualities of health. "Well being, as succinctly defined by Daniel Siegel, has the following dimensions:

- life energy and vitality
- stability and flexibility
- coherence and adaptability
- balance of autonomy and connectedness"[cliv]
- engagement in acts of service

Well-being is significantly strengthened by time well spent in acknowledging and celebrating healthy capacities, successes, and growth.

Well-being, to state the obvious, is not just important for those we serve. "To be able to assist our clients to integrate and free their natural drive toward maximum complexity, we ourselves need to have developed the following capacities:

- to self-reflect
- to attune to another
- to hold the other in our hearts and minds in a loving gentle way"[clv]

Referrals for Psychological Help

For helping professionals (such as massage therapists, body workers, coaches, and medical practitioners) who do not have extensive psychotherapy training or responsibility for working with serious psychological issues, here is a bit of guidance for helping to determine whether a client might need psychological help.

As a touchstone for what psychological health can be, here are some qualities present in people with consistent, reliable self-image.[clvi]

1) A capacity to experience and express a wide range of feelings deeply, and these feelings are appropriate to their current life situation.
2) A capacity to expect appropriate entitlements and a sense of confidence about their past history.
3) Successful functioning is durable, transportable, and coherent.
4) A capacity for self-activation and assertion. They have dreams and goals. They take the necessary steps to achieve these goals and defend their dreams when they are challenged.
5) An ability to acknowledge their own self-worth and have resilient coping abilities.
6) An ability to soothe painful feelings and make choices about what will be more or less painful.
7) An ability to make and stick to commitments despite obstacles and setbacks.
8) Creativity: the ability to replace old, familiar patterns of problem-solving with new and equally or more successful ones, cope with loss, and adjust to new life circumstances.
9) Intimacy: the ability to express their true self fully and honestly in close relationship with minimal anxiety and little fear of abandonment or engulfment.
10) The ability to be alone and be enough.
11) Continuity of self: a core that persists through time and space. The "I" of one experience is the same as the "I" of another experience.

Any lacks or deficits in the above qualities may be a reason to refer.

Handling Emotional Triggering

Here is some guidance for Handling Emotional Triggering and Catharsis provided by Mukara Meredith. [clvii]

If your client gets so activated or triggered that they cannot be present for the kind of work that you do, you can assist them by staying connected, calm, and present. In addition:

- **Stay Body-centered**
  Focus on sensation and avoid analysis.
  "What are you noticing in your body? What happens next? Does it move through your whole body? What specifically is the sensation?"

- **Go Slowly**
  Slow things down through your pacing and willingness to take charge. This will reverse the acceleration of overwhelming experience.
  "Let's slow things down now. We have all the time we need. I will help you take your time with this. Let's stay in contact with eyes open."

- **Find the appropriate physical distance**
  They may need more space or more contact. Ask them.

- **Focus on Grounding**
  Attend to lower areas of body—"feet and seat."
  Encourage downward movement of energy. Pushing through the feet and legs is helpful for grounding.

- **Reconnect to resources and support**
  "You are not alone now. It's over, you made it. What got you through all that? You are here now and you are okay. You have support now."

- **Loop or Stitch**
  Connect to impulses and support their fulfillment and completion.
  "What lets you know you are okay just now? If your body could have anything, what would it want right now? Feel that and notice where you feel good, or open in your body."

Handling emotional triggering, paying attention to making timely and appropriate referrals and taking time to complete sessions skillfully are right uses of your role power and will help you earn your client's trust.

Self-Study: Reviewing

What is the practical part about the process of terminating and making referrals?   What is the vulnerable part?

How does the power differential increase the complexity and/or possibility for misunderstanding?

Dimension Four: Be Skillful

Topics covered in this section:
Feedback
Self-Care
Influence, Values, Diversity
Leadership & Power Dynamics
Challenges
Soul Work & World Service

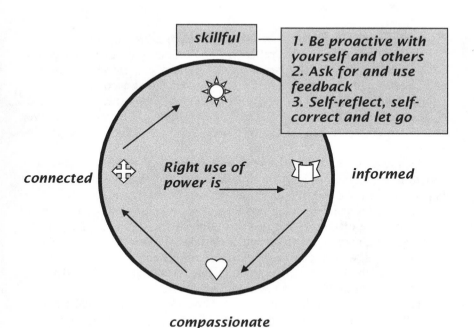

Focus on Wisdom
- *Right Use of Power is Skillful*
- *Dimension Four is about Wisdom.*

  - *Thinking and behaving pro-actively to prevent harm and promote well-being*

  - *Knowing your values and being sensitive to diversity*

  - *Practicing and modeling a ethic of compassion*

  - *Giving precedence to good self-care in service relationships and in your life*

  - *Being familiar with some power dynamics and leadership styles*

  - *Making real your intentions*

  - *Asking for and utilizing the resource of feedback*

  - *Dancing the dance with precision and grace.*

  - *Connecting with the largest context of world service*

Power Spiral—Topics in the Wisdom Dimension
Skillful use of power is a reflection of a refined level of personal and soul development. Skillful use of power requires experience, awareness and understanding of the ever-unfolding dynamics that accompany power issues. It calls for learning how and when to lead and follow, when to take charge, and when to let go. From this empowerment, a larger perspective and vision emerges. Skillful use of power is the full use of one's gifts in service.

This level of ethics involves an understanding of power that can't be coded into rules. It is a level of consciousness and awareness of self and impact that is at the forefront of the evolution of consciousness.

This section is a launching pad for further evolution of wisdom about the skillful use of power. We make an authentic assessment of potential challenges, vulnerabilities to particular mistakes. By becoming clear about our challenges, we can take the additional step of being pro-actively aware and alert for these fuzzy edges. Asking for, receiving, giving, and using feedback about our edges is a key to empowerment.

Topics included in this section are oriented around additional themes: influence, values, and diversity issues, leadership and power dynamics, and self-care as an ethical issue. The section ends with a look at ethics as soul work and world service.

Three Skills and Wisdoms

Be pro-active with yourself and others

The power for health and the power for harm resides in the quality and integrity in relationship. By thinking and acting proactively you, you can wisely and skillfully prevent harm and also teach others about using their power better.

Ask for and use feedback well

The most valuable skill for using power wisely and well is feedback. Using feedback well keep your relationships current and empathic.

Self-reflect, self-correct and let go

Staying connected, resolving difficulties, and repairing the relationship as soon as possible will usually prevent conflicts from escalating. The process of using self-reflection to self-correct and refine will increase your effectiveness and satisfaction.

Barriers and Resources to Wisdom

Barriers to wisdom and empowerment seem to center around fear of one's potential for goodness. "If I do well this time, people will expect me to be perfect." "I don't want to be seen as arrogant." "What I'm doing is just a little thing, not skillful use of power." "If I'm powerful, I'll cause harm." "I'm not strong enough." " If I use my power, I'll be visible and get attacked." These attitudes are reflected in habits of disowning power, not fully showing up, over-focusing on personal wounds and suffering, not taking a stand. Participants have discovered such things as: "I don't have to wait until I'm not scared to begin. I can use my fear to remind myself of my integrity and sensitivity." "I will use my power to create my life." "I am now confident that I can use my power with love." "I am learning to recognize when to let go of something."

Resources include the lessons of lived experience, openness to feedback from others, self-care activities, a lively and engaging attitude of curiosity, and capacity for wisdom and compassion.

Power Spiral Layer

This fourth dimension layer of the spiral, is a wisdom layer. Culled from much research about indigenous tribes, Angeles Arrien,[clviii] a Basque anthropologist, discerned that there were four elements common to these tribes. These elements formed a kind of prescription for living the good life. They also relate to the focus of each dimension: Information, Self, Relationship, Wisdom.

Showing up is the place to begin. The sun begins its daily journey (from our perspective) in the East. So much new and familiar **Information** is available. Fully showing up is more of a challenge than it might seem. Showing up as a caregiver means being centered, resourced, and available during sessions.

Paying attention to what has heart and meaning is surely about knowing your **Self**, your history, your beliefs, your values, your gifts, so that you can use the power of them benevolently and for yourself and others.

Telling and hearing the truth without shame or blame is most definitely connected to **Relationships**. The truth will set you free, and giving and receiving truthful feedback will fine-tune, clarify, and deepen relationships. Truth telling can be skillfully done without the isolating, de-resourcing and escalating effects of shame and blame.

Being open to outcome, not attached to it. This is the **Wisdom** of the North where a sense of the greater mystery and faith in influences and unfoldings that we cannot yet see, offers a letting go of effort. Right use of power often involves letting go of your personal image or need for a particular outcome. Non-attachment opens the doorway to creative solutions and directions that could not be seen through the attachments.

This spiral holds wisdom and guidance for both personal and professional wise and skillful use of power.

Four-Fold Path[clix]

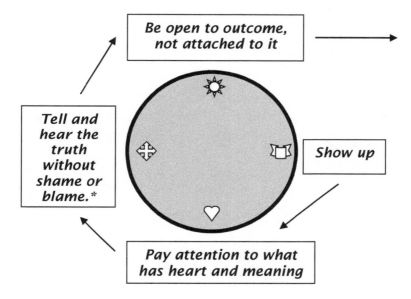

* Wording changes with Arrien's permission, from original — "Tell the truth without blame or judgment."

"The power within—the more you give, the more you have to give—will be our source when coal and oil are long gone, and atoms are left to spin in peace." —*Gary Snyder* [clx]

Feedback

Standing in your power, staying in your heart. [clxi]

Feedback is an investment in relationship. [clxii]

Right use of power is a life-long engagement with understanding more about your impact on others.

Story: The most challenging feedback Karen ever received was also the most helpful. Several of her students told her that she was so patient and flexible that her classes felt slow and "draggy." Specifically, they had noticed that she would say something definitive, like "Now we're going to...," and then add, "or does anyone have something else to say first?" This created confusion. This feedback was painful to hear, but when Karen worked on being more directive and trusted her own sense of what was next, classes had more momentum and students relaxed into her leadership.

Feedback is any response, negative or positive, that is given to someone else about the impact of their behavior. For example—feedback could be about skillfulness, ideas, presentation, style, or impact. Feedback is a specific form of communication that is deliberate, considerate, specific, and somewhat detached. Feedback provides an opportunity to learn how others perceive your behavior and to let others know how they are perceived. It is aimed at fostering more awareness rather than getting another to change in accordance with your wishes and/or perceptions.

Seeking and using feedback will help you

- encourage open and authentic communication
- keep your relationships current and alive
- learn more about yourself and your impact
- prevent problems from developing
- handle problems after they occur

- deepen relationships
- clarify relationship issues
- fine tune alignment between your intentions and your impact

Skillfulness with power is learned through reflecting on your experiences—both the successful and unsuccessful ones, through paying fine-tuned attention to how your clients are responding to both your methods and your ways of relating, and through increasing your understanding of power dynamics. Getting feedback from your clients, colleagues, and environment about the impact of your use of your power is an art and a skill.

Like the concepts of ethics and power, feedback seems to have an automatic negative connotation. When you hear "Can I give you some feedback?" do you brace yourself for something bad? The first thing to do is to reframe feedback to include both positive and negative information. It is also helpful not to immediately categorize what you hear as positive or negative.[clxiii] The other helpful reframe is understanding and feeling feedback in the context of deepening and improving relationships. As my friend Amina Knowlan puts it, *"Feedback is an investment in relationship."* This idea shifts the focus from behavior to relationship. It is when in respectful relationship that we are most likely to be able to use feedback to learn and grow.

Many years ago, in a Sensitivity Training[clxiv] program, I learned about JoHari's Window. This is a little map of Self that is directly related to how feedback increases your self-knowledge. It looks like a window with four panes in it. It illuminates four kinds of information we have about ourselves and about others. There are things that are:

Self	*Other*	
Known to Self and unknown to Others (such as your mother's middle name)	Known to Other and known to Self (such as your name)	*Known*
Unknown to Self and known to Others (such as a familiar and unconscious gesture)	Unknown to Self and unknown to Others (such as the unconscious contents of your psyche	*Unknown*

Curiosity about your impact and asking for feedback can assist you in increasing the amount of self-knowledge that is available. In other words, you can lower the horizontal bar in JoHari's Window.

In my experience, facility with the four aspects of the art of feedback is the **single most important skill** to develop for right use of power and influence in effective and satisfying service. **Feedback, both positive and critical, can be encouraging and then well-used when offered and received with compassion and respect. The most important idea is to endeavor to offer your feedback in a way that it can best be received, and in a way that you stay in relationship.** Ascertaining how your words can best be received by the individual you are offering them to is a high-level skill. Staying in touch with your desire and ability to make a good investment in this relationship is the attitude that will get you to the gold.

1. Asking for feedback

For many people, the idea that they can take charge of how and when they receive feedback by asking for it directly is a new and empowering idea. Engaging pro-actively with people about how you affect them will also do much to clarify, deepen and enrich your professional and collegial relationships.

- Be pro-active.
- Ask often. Feedback keeps relationships alive, interesting, healthy, and engaged.
- Be specific in your request: *"I'm curious about how you experience my _____(name a behavior.)"*
- Include in your request information about how you would like the feedback to be offered: timing, pacing, balance of positive and negative, how much.
- Ask for feedback about new behavior right away.
- Get feedback from multiple sources about issues of particular concern to you.

You may want to ask for feedback from clients when:
- You don't understand a response (*"I'm wondering if your lateness today has something to do with your feelings about how our sessions are going?"*)
- You are curious (*"I'm curious about how you're feeling about the work we're doing together. I'd like some feedback."*)

- You sense some kind of problem (*"I'm sensing that there might be some kind of problem here and I'd like to attend to it."*)
- You want to repair the relationship (*"What could we do to repair the relationship?"*)

2. Giving feedback

Your skillfulness and sensitivity in giving feedback is a big factor in how well your client or colleague can hear and use your input. Being guided by compassion and respect is the most important factor and these things can support your intention to be helpful.

- Ask the receiver about their willingness to receive feedback and their availability to take it in.
- Be compassionate, authentic, and courageous.
- Be specific and concrete, using examples from the present or recent past.
- Be direct and speak slowly.
- Keep it simple and spacious.
- Identify interpretations: *"I'm imagining that..."*
- Speak about concrete behavior rather than personality.
- Balance positive and negative feedback
- Track for when the receiver may have heard enough.
- Suggest a specific, behavioral change or other option.
- Don't use positive feedback as a way to get the receiver to change or to like you.
- Don't be attached to the outcome.

3. Receiving feedback

People need truth linked with kindness. In a supportive environment they can hear and respond to "difficult to hear" information in a positive way.

- Relax and take a breath.
- Take responsibility for setting the parameters: timing, pacing, how much, what kind?
- Be actively receptive, not defensive.
- Listen and delay trying to explain yourself.
- Ask for specific example(s) in addition to perception. Ask for clarification.

- Be curious about yourself, your impact, and your state of mind while receiving feedback.
- Acknowledge and restate the feedback as you understand it.
- Receive feedback as a gift affording you an opportunity to learn and grow.
- Respond to feedback in a way that encourages future communication.
- Have an open mind and don't assume you know what the giver means.

4. Using feedback

Using feedback is an application process that goes beyond receiving it.

- If it is something new and previously outside your awareness, ask several others about their perceptions.
- Give challenging feedback some space and time before deciding how to use it.
- Understand that feedback is also about the giver. It may be both an offering and a projection.
- Try a piece of feedback on before deciding on its accuracy or usefulness.
- Keep what is useful and with a breath of kindness, blow the rest away.
- Link specific feedback with a behavioral change that addresses it and actively and deliberately experiment with this change.
- Be appreciative and let the giver know how you are using their feedback.

Feedback Challenges

Here are some challenges related to using feedback.

A. Fear of causing pain

People often worry about hurting others when offering authentic, yet critical and difficult to hear feedback. It's important to be in the other person's moccasins, when giving feedback. Empathy and sensitivity, compassion and connection, and a level of truthfulness that people can hear and gratefully use, is important.

B. Vulnerability

Asking for or receiving feedback is courageous but can feel vulnerable. As my friend Karen Blicher says, "*Remember Star Trek, well, I have an automatic 'shields up' response to feedback. Absolutely nothing is going to get in."* Receiving feedback is a vulnerable activity and often triggers dysfunctional, automatic responses that include:

- taking feedback as the whole truth
- withdrawing and de-resourcing in shame
- deflecting all information--both positive and negative
- dismissing or denying
- taking refuge in confusion
- shutting down

Pro-actively asking for feedback is a powerful way to choose when you need another's perspective.

C. Feedback loop
Leaders and people in power positions are especially likely to get out of the normal feedback loop and get either no feedback or only positive or skewed feedback. Students, clients, employees, generally have an investment in being liked, valued, and well-treated by those in a power differential role. They may feel, or actually be at risk when they need to give negative feedback. Those in a up-power role may also need to be active about encouraging and responding sensitively to all kinds of feedback.

D. Character feedback and process feedback
Sometimes it is hard to distinguish between feedback that is valuable and that which criticizes your character or style. Your character or style may not be possible or desirable to change. For example, "Your teaching style is too spacious," or "Your voice is too gentle," or "You aren't personal enough," or, "You're too abrupt." It is often more important to acknowledge the feedback and address the response to you as a relationship dynamic to understand and work with.
Story: Gail's client was critical about the slow pacing of sessions and frequently wanted Gail to just jump in and direct. She gave this process feedback to Gail. When Gail responded by moving to a faster pace, Gail's client was surprised to discover that the faster pace frightened her and that she actually needed to go very slowly in order to feel safe enough. In this case, process feedback moved into therapeutic character work. Working with the dynamic of her habitual impatience was very productive.

E. Too much caution

We are blessed with an innate impulse to learn and grow. We long to know how we impact others. When not feeling ashamed or embarrassed about not being perfect, we can be excited and empowered by feedback that enables us to change something that was causing limitations or unnecessary suffering. Putting too much reliance on a "formula" for feedback, we can become stilted or flat. Take courage in your authenticity.

F. Differentiating Feedback

There is a fine, but useful, distinction between feedback used to connect through similarities and feedback used to connect through differences.[clxv] Feedback like, "I understand and agree," or "I would have done the same thing," or, "My version of that is," connects. Feedback like, "I see things differently," or "I would have. . . .", or "We have a difference here. From my different perspective, I suggest. . . .," or "Have you thought about something very different?" differentiates. It is helpful to be clear about when you are agreeing and when you are differentiating. Differentiating is a more conceptually-friendly word than disagreeing.

G. Using feedback creatively and well

Story: As a teacher, I have a number of times received feedback from large groups that the Right Use of Power program was too slow and that I spoke too slowly. I have used this feedback to rearrange the curriculum, use a power point, speak a bit faster, rev up the pacing, but still I was getting the "too slow" feedback from some people in each large group. In talking it over with some colleagues and getting beyond my defensiveness, I realized that it wasn't so much about my speeding up (not my nature) but about encouraging my students to slow down. I needed to explain a bit more about experiential education and learning ethics from the inside out. Most ethical decision-making happens from the inside, in ordinary moments using our curiosity, integrity, skills, gut and attunement to the relationship. I needed to invite them to give themselves a break from the rush of their lives and slow down to get the most from the program. This was a surprising and productive insight. Using feedback well doesn't always mean doing what is suggested or implied.

H. Assuming we know what is going on with the other

It's a simple and human thing. We feel empathy and we assume we know what the other person is thinking and feeling. Yvonne Agazarian,[clxvi] a well-know group process trainer, has a simple recommendation for getting feedback about assumptions. You simply ask the other person if you can do a mind-read with them. If they say yes, you tell them what you are imagining they are thinking or feeling particularly as it relates to you. Then you ask them to tell you what is accurate and what is not. Then you reflect back what you heard. Simple, direct, clarifying, often relieving.

I. Sometimes you just get dumped on or projected on

It happens. We might be in an up-power role, or in a down-power role. Someone dumps a lot of verbal and energetic negative criticism. They don't notice how you are being impacted. They don't seem to care about being effective. They are just letting you have it. My friend Charna,[clxvii] has some good guidance, especially for when you are in an up-power role and must maintain your dignity and be respectful.

1. Step aside and call out your observer self
2. Watch it
3. Mine it, shake it out, look for the nugget of truth
4. Work with the nugget
5. Respond to the giver

J. Further insights

Amina Knowlan, a group leadership trainer, offers some further insights. *Feedback is not a demand for change. It may be followed by a request for change, but the feedback itself is just data. Conflict, in my experience, is often a hyper-charged backlog of undelivered feedback. By the time we deliver the feedback, there is such a build-up of dissatisfaction that it often comes with an intention and tone that sounds like a demand for change or even a threat.*

If I am giving you feedback about the impact of your behavior on me, I am not blaming you, or making you responsible for that impact. I am offering data about your impact on me as a way of opening the communication between us and improving our relationship. Feedback might be thought of as a way of "lubricating" the channels of communication between us. If, as Desmond Tutu says, 'We can only go forward together,' then feedback becomes a way of lending each other a hand. If we really grasped this concept that so fundamentally expresses the assumption of interconnectedness, then how could we not want to receive feedback about our impact? Why would we spend so much time defending our intentions rather than just staying curious about our impact?[clxviii]

K. Session Feedback Forms

Psychotherapists have found that asking for frequent feedback from clients to be so helpful in refining and deepening their psychotherapeutic relationships that they use very simple written feedback instruments that take a few minutes to complete. These include questions such as: *"On a scale of 1-10, how helpful was this session? What was most helpful? Was there anything that was unhelpful? What did you learn? What helped this new learning to happen?" Do you feel you are making progress in relation to your therapy goals? If not, what specifically do you want to address? Name a measurable and do-able action step you can take now.*[clxix]

Self-Study: Feedback

Awareness and feedback, like a Mobius strip, continually loop around and support each other.

1. Take a breath and relax and turn your awareness inside and let your unconscious offer you a memory of a time when you received some feedback that was difficult to hear. Notice the details of your experience and response: thoughts, sensations, emotions, images, impulses, and automatic habits. Now experiment with giving yourself enough distance to receive whatever is true about this communication and let go of the rest.

Take another breath, relax, and let yourself be curious about the effect(s) of your power on others. Ask a friend or colleague for some specific feedback using the suggestions listed earlier about asking for feedback and for receiving feedback. If you can't think of anything specific to ask about, just say: "Tell me an affect I have on you." Another interesting question would be: "Tell me a way you experience my use of power as similar to yours, and a way it is different from yours." Or, "Could you give me an example of a time when you felt I used my power well?" "Or a time when my use of power was ineffective?"

When you get some particularly challenging or helpful feedback, reflect on a specific way that you could get support in working with this information, and ask for help.

2.   Try this self-study with a partner…Each of you think of whatever would be your most dreaded feedback, i.e. what you most fear hearing. (Like, *"You're no good at this and it's hopeless."*) Partner A says this feedback to Partner B. Partner B notices and responds with habitual pattern (i.e. shuts down, blames the other, feels guilty, etc.). Experience the impact of this response. Now Partner A offers the same feedback and Partner B finds and tries out another response that would be more likely to lead toward clarity, resolution, and relationship repair. Notice the impact and reverse roles.

3.   Practice asking for feedback. Keep in mind that feedback at its best is an investment in relationship.   Ask a friend or colleague about anything you are curious about. Or ask a general question such as, "tell me an effect my use of power has on you." Asking offers you an opportunity to be pro-active.

When teaching the skill of feedback, I ask students to partner up and engage with each other in a series of feedback questions and statements. They switch partners with each question or stay with the same partner to go deeper with their investment in that one relationship. I ask all or some of these questions.   After each question I ask the students to notice what affect this has had on their relationship.   (Deeper, closer, richer, more present, is the usual answer.) I also ask how accurate and how interesting the feedback they get is even when they don't know each other well. (Surprisingly accurate is the usual answer.)   Here are some questions to experiment with in addition to the ones in #1 above.

Asking for feedback: *Tell me an affect I have on you.*
Receiving feedback: *Something I notice about your use of power is*
_____*.*

Possibly challenging feedback: *Something that might be challenging for me in working with you is* _____*.*
Receiving feedback: *A wish I have for you in the use of your power is*
_____*.*

Using feedback: *What do I wish for myself? What insight or understanding am I taking away from this feedback?*

Self-Care

Sitting in my seat with my seat belt fastened on dozens of airplanes, I have half-heard the flight attendant say, "Put your oxygen mask on yourself first before putting it on your child." On my last flight, I pondered this. Of course, when you are in the service role, you need literally to make sure you are breathing or you will be of no help to your clients.

Helping professionals tend to focus their energies and attention toward service and care of others to the detriment of their own care. So committed to service and healing, they frequently forget that when they are "burned out," their clients won't be getting the level of professional care that the caregivers are capable of offering.

Self-care attitudes

It is easy to feel that somehow the chair is sitting on you, rather than you sitting on the chair. The meditation masters know this well. Here is a self-reflection activity that will help you explore your relationship with self-care. Turn your awareness inside and notice your experience when you imagine hearing the words: "It's okay to take care of yourself." Are any of these feelings or beliefs familiar to you? How do you stop yourself from getting adequate self-care?

- *"I don't have time to exercise, or _____."*
- *"My clients need me."*
- *"I need to work more to make it financially."*
- *"My sessions always run over because I want clients to get as much as possible, and I don't get the 10 minutes break that I need."*
- *"My service work comes first and play is self-indulgence or laziness."*
- *"There are too many demands on me—work, relationship, children, financial needs... and I come last, it seems."*
- *"Time is just not on my side."*

- *"I get more and more stressed and accommodate with less and less sleep until I collapse."*
- *"The only way I get to stop is when I get sick."*
- *"If I take some time off, there's so much to do to catch up when I get back that it's not worth it."*
- *"I feel ashamed when I feel needy. It's just not okay."*
- *"I feel my clients pain so much that I sometimes get overwhelmed and take on their hopelessness."*
- *"My needs are so small compared to those of others in my care."*
- *"I have a great practice. I don't feel a need for supervision or peer support."*
- *"I have a strong ethic of service."*
- *"When I've gotten myself to the point of being exhausted, I make it worse by feeling ashamed that I haven't taken care of myself and then I try to cover it up even more…it becomes a vicious cycle."*

Inadequate self-care results

Self-care is a significant ethical issue because:

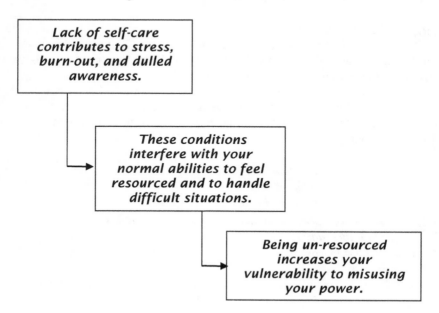

Lack of self-care contributes to stress, burn-out, and dulled awareness.

These conditions interfere with your normal abilities to feel resourced and to handle difficult situations.

Being un-resourced increases your vulnerability to misusing your power.

Note: the term resourced means being connected to and supported by personal resources, e.g. centeredness, confidence, compassion, education and training, supervision, empowerment, social network.

Recent brain and energy research offers very specific data about the impact of stress on the brain. When stressed, blood flows away from the brain and into our extremities, in preparation for "fight or flight" which leaves us less able to be connected and creatively respond to challenging situations.[clxx]

Take a minute to recall—and we have all had these moments—a time when a client arrived and you were tired, emotionally exhausted, burned out, stressed… What is your experience like?

Results of lack of self-care include:

- impaired judgment
- dulled alertness and attention
- reduced warmth and generosity
- increased defensiveness
- more easily triggered annoyance, frustration, or anger
- over-confidence
- murky boundaries
- over or under involvement
- lack of compassion or over-compassion
- decreased sensitivity to transferences
- illness or burn-out
- resentment
- inadequate record keeping

Right use of power are uses of power that prevent, reduce, and repair harm to clients *and Self,* and that promote experienced and sustainable well-being for clients *and for Self.* Self-less service is often thought of as the ideal. More truly what is needed is self-full service, or service from a full use of self. When thinking about ethical behavior and ethical attitudes, *Right Use of Power* is about not causing harm to ourselves as well as our clients.

Misusing power against Self

There are many subtle ways that we misuse our power with ourselves.

Failing to prevent or reduce harm to ourselves

For example, getting so overwhelmed or over-worked that you develop debilitating symptoms of caregiver burn-out.

Failing to repair harm to ourselves

For example, being overly self-critical, having unreasonable expectations, lacking self-compassion, feeling ashamed and not attending to healing these.

Failing to promote our own well-being

Undervaluing your work and effectiveness, not finding nourishment in your work, and not confidently owning your role power.

Self-care and the 150% principle

"Yikes! How do you adequately take care of yourself when your job requires you to bear 150% responsibility for those in your care? I overwork already," I am often asked by students and readers. So in one of my programs we addressed this question and came up with a list.

Taking care of yourself while staying in the role of greater responsibility:

- know you can't fix people
- apologize
- accurately assess the 150%
- let yourself grieve
- forgive
- take down-time
- use supervision and peer support
- remember to take you role off
- be careful about what phone calls you take
- discern when you have done enough and then let go

The neuroscience of well-being

Neuroscience continues to influence our understanding of how to be good, happy and high-functioning human beings. Dr. Richie Davidson is a neuroscientist who is researching healthy minds at the Center for Investigating Healthy Minds. His research has identified four qualities that contribute to Well-Being and that are influenced by discipline and training. These are:[clxxi]

  1. *Resilience: The ability to recover rapidly from adversity*

2. *Focus on Positive Emotion: The ability to be aware of thoughts and feelings and move the mind away from excessive negativity and toward uplifting emotions like Love, Joy, Compassion, Gratitude and Empathy*
3. *Generosity: The ability to practice the art of sincere and genuine giving.*
4. *Attention: The ability to stay in the present moment and not engage in mind wandering*

Strengthening Resilience

Resilience is the ability to bounce back--to cope successfully with adversity or risk and to learn new skills from doing so. Increasing your resilience is an essential foundation for self-care. Practicing the self-care strategies mentioned in this chapter will contribute to increasing your resilience. The image of a tree--deeply rooted and yet able to be flexible even in strong wind, comes to mind. Another way to increase your resilience is to go deeper in the power spiral. In the east, clarify and refine how you receive and use guidance, in the south, delve into more self-awareness, in the west, practice staying connected and non-defensive, and in the north, get more grounded in your wisdom and skill. Resilience: standing in your strength while staying in your heart.

Fostering Gratitude

Fostering gratitude by noticing and appreciating the positive aspects of life contributes remarkably to a sense of well-being. In fact in a study of 400 people, 40% of whom had sleep problems, researchers found that grateful people slept better, stayed asleep longer and had less difficulty falling back asleep.[clxxii] Gratitude is an emotion and it is also a habit that can be developed. Practice by starting and ending your day with gratitude, being thankful for simple things, looking for the positive in the negative, and saying thank you.[clxxiii]

My friend, Anna Cox is the founder of Compassion Works For All, a non-profit organization that provides resources for prisoners and helps them accept responsibility for their lives and cope with loss and the difficulties of life in prison. In a meditation session on gratefulness in a prison in Little Rock, Arkansas, here are some of the things the men said to each other about their gratitude: *"You were the first person to speak to me when I came to prison." "When I was having such a hard time the other day, you were there for me and really helped me out of a bad time."* A white Christian hugged an African American Muslim saying, *"You are my brother from another mother."* Anna says, "after each person had received their round of gratitude, I asked them to just feel what was given to them. They did, deeply, and they saw that their lives do matter."[clxxiv]

Being Pro-Active

Understanding your vulnerabilities is a powerful piece of self-care. Knowing, for example, that it is "over-the-top" important to you to be liked by your clients, you will be attuned to your tendency to resist saying something therapeutic to your clients that might also be challenging. You can then "catch" yourself and self-correct, thus preventing possible harm. For another example, if you know yourself to have poor time boundaries, you can pro-actively begin ending the session a few minutes earlier than usual.

Modeling self-care

One of the most potent ways to use power and influence to promote well-being is modeling right use of power for our clients. Modeling self-care by, for example, keeping good time boundaries, taking breaks during your work day, keeping an uncluttered office, and not over scheduling demonstrates your everyday practice of honoring your own needs.

Story. *In one of my sessions, I was feeling quite upset with myself because I was too tired and was having difficulty keeping my eyes open. After some minutes of valiantly fighting it, I said, "I'm really sorry, but I'm feeling sleepy. This isn't about you. I am going to take a few minutes break to wake myself up." When I came back in a few minutes, my client had teared up, saying, "What you did really touched me. I can't tell you how many times I've been there trying not to fall asleep and feeling guilty. It never occurred to me that I could be so honest and do something to wake up. I'm so relieved to know that you take care of yourself. And it wasn't a problem. In fact, while you were gone, I had an interesting insight."*

Self-Care Package

Good self-care is a rich package involving more than just getting enough sleep. Self-care involves taking care of yourself both within the context of your helping relationships and in your life outside your work.[clxxv]

Self-Assessment Chart

The primary question is: **What does it take for me to show up for my clients in a way I feel good about?** Give yourself an opportunity to look at your self-care personally and within the therapeutic relationship. *Rate yourself on a scale of 1—10 with 10 meaning that you are very good at this aspect of self-care.*

Balance		
1. Maintaining an appropriate work-load	1 ←————→	10
2. Creating diversity of expressive, recreational, and spiritual activities	1 ←————→	10
3. Developing the ability to both savor and serve	1 ←————→	10
4. Setting a high priority on self-care	1 ←————→	10
5. Attending to your inner balance	1 ←————→	10
Rest		
6. Getting enough rest and retreat time	1 ←————→	10
7. Planning ahead for times of renewal	1 ←————→	10
8. Allowing for goof off time	1 ←————→	10
9. Getting adequate physical exercise	1 ←————→	10
10. Being kind and compassionate toward yourself.	1 ←————→	10
Satisfaction		
11. Approaching clients with an attitude of curiosity—savoring & being nourished by their essential qualities; feeling gratitude	1 ←————→	10
12 Appreciating the value and importance of your professional offerings	1 ←————→	10
13. Finding novelty in daily routine and resting in the ease of familiar skillfulness	1 ←————→	10
14. Feeling a sense of inner satisfaction and pleasure in your work	1 ←————→	10
15. Staying in touch with your desire and vision for service.	1 ←————→	10
Support		
16. Using supervision and personal support	1 ←————→	10
17. Keeping appropriate records, disclosure forms, and malpractice insurance	1 ←————→	10
18. Knowing, accepting, and accommodating for your limitations	1 ←————→	10
19. Seeking and using feedback	1 ←————→	10
20. Accessing continuing education that is inspiring, informative, and stimulating	1 ←————→	10

Here's a little more background on several of the items listed in the self-assessment.

Item #3. Serving and Savoring

This quote from E. B. White got me to thinking. *"I awake each morning torn between my desire to save the world and my desire to savor the world. This makes it very difficult to plan my day."*[clxxvi] Spending some time walking from one pole to the other in my living room, I got clear that, of course, the choice is not between one or the other—saving or savoring—but finding service in savoring and savoring in service. Taken to an extreme, savoring becomes an ineffective and flat self-indulgence, and taken to the other extreme, serving becomes a desperate and burned-out saving the world. Finding ways to savor—your experiences, beauty, integrity—while you are serving will add richness, nourishment and satisfaction to your experience of service; and finding ways to serve will add meaning and depth to your appreciation of life.

Item #4. Self-care as a priority

A student puts it this way: *"I just didn't get the ethics of this until now. Self-care never even got on my priority list. It was like a luxury or a reward for over-working. Now I understand how my lack of self-care seriously disrupts my ability to be present with my clients. So my question is going to be—'What does it take for me to show up for my clients in a way that I feel good about?' For me at the most basic level that means having gotten enough sleep, exercise, and meditation."* [clxxvii]

Item #5. Attending to your inner polarity balance

4. Between the extremes of attachment and apathy

3. Between the extremes of projection and introjection

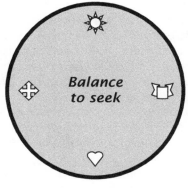

Balance to seek

1. Between the extremes of ignorance and overwhelm

2. Between the extremes of unconsciousness and self-absorption

Balance is essential in self-care. The Power Spiral describes a kind of balance to seek that is endemic to each of the quadrants of the spiral.

The task in the **Guided use of power (1)** is to manage being open to receiving relevant, important, and current information from within and from without. "Without" includes other people and various forms of written material. Being too open can result in overwhelm, confusion, despair. Being too closed can result in mistakes that could have been avoided.

The task in the **Conscious use of power (2)** is to learn to be vulnerable and knowledgeable about your history, habits, and woundings and yet not so focused on them that you cannot be emotionally available to attend to the relationships at hand.

The task of the **Responsible use of power (3)** is to find a balance that allows you to take responsibility for what is yours—not taking too much responsibility and de-resourcing in shame (introjection) or too little responsibility by blaming it on the other (projection).

The task of the **Wise use of power (4)** is learning when to persist and when to let go. A wise leader knows when to move forward and when to move back, how to pick out what is most important and let the rest be, how to be the banks of the river, and how to avoid becoming stuck in over-attachment or so apathetic that followers do not feel guided.

Item #10. Being kind and compassionate toward yourself

Secondary Traumatic Stress refers to the traumatic stress that can be experienced by caregivers as they work with clients in pain and suffering. Sometimes this is referred to as "compassion fatigue." It is often unrecognized and under-attended. B. Hudnell Stamm writes: *"Secondary Traumatic Stress makes [a demand] on us: to depart from believing in the illusion that we are protected from other's pain by scientific postures and our 'white coats.' I would not suggest that we leave objectivity behind, but that we recognize that our personal passions drive our desires to do this work and our training and good supervision—of our clinical work, or research, or our teaching—helps us keep our balance and objectivity. Objectivity and flintiness are not a guarantee of our training. Nor should they be. The capacity for compassion and empathy seem to be at the core of our ability to do the work and at the core of our ability to be wounded by the work."*[clxxviii]

Item #11. Approaching clients with an attitude of curiosity— savoring and being nourished by their essential qualities; feeling gratitude

Replacing an anxious "having to know everything" with an attitude of curiosity and attention to what is happening, can bring more ease and healing receptiveness for both you and your clients.

Ron Kurtz calls savoring "non-egocentric nourishment." [clxxix] This is the ability to be nourished by the essential qualities of your clients. This is significantly different from ego pleasure of being a good therapist or making a good intervention or having a great insight. It is a kind of ordinary and transcendent nourishment. It might start with the enjoyment of curiosity and discovery. It might come through seeing the vulnerability or suffering of the other. You are searching for the universal, for the grace and beauty, for some essential good you can see in your client and finding some way you can start to let that fill you up. Your clients will feel your delight and appreciation and not only will you feel more satisfied and less tired, but your practice will be helping your clients learn more self-compassion and appreciation.

Item #16. Asking for support

For helping professionals, asking for help is often felt as a sign of weakness or inadequacy. Think of asking for help as an art. As a colleague said, *"Be efficient with your needs. Tell people what you need. Teach people how to leave you alone if they are bugging you. Teach people how to please you if they are taking advantage of you. Teaching can be kind and gentle. The point is to make your needs known in a way they can be met."*[clxxx] When you ask for help and the answer is "no," ask the person, "If you can't do this, what could you do?" or "What part of what I am asking for could you do." When others ask you for help, practice responding with what, however small, you CAN do, rather than pained excuses for what you can't do.

Item #18. Limitations

Most often the focus of personal development is on improving in areas of weakness. This is one part of becoming more skillful. But there is another half of skillfulness. That is accepting and accommodating to limitations. Limitations are important. We all have them. If you are not good at remembering details, it may be more skillful to take time to make clear notes after a session, than trying to remember things better and getting upset when you don't. If you know you have a hard time with time boundaries, it may be more skillful to accept this and tell your clients that you are setting your watch for 10 minutes before the end of the session so that it will beep as a reminder to both of you of the time boundary, rather than stressing about going over-time.

"It's not easy to be sure that being true to yourself is worth the trouble, but we do know that it is our sacred duty."
—*Florida Scott Maxwell*[clxxxi]

Never be too busy for three breaths. Three breaths is key to everything.
—*C.B.*

Situational Ethics

I told a lie on Monday
when the morning sun rose fogless
for the first time in weeks.
I said I was busy, already booked,
seeing emergency clients
who had called the night before,
desperate for light on their situations.
It was almost the truth,
like a half of a moon,
the hidden part being
that I was the one desperate
for light, the one busy
with a need to dream,
my body spread out on the sand
under a tent of blue,
my only appointment
with the ocean herself,
waiting patiently
to cleanse my guilt,
her briny sting forgiving every lie
ever told in the name of saving
oneself from that other deluge
that can drown the soul
if you are not careful,
the tsunami of hours
too generously promised to others
that comes crashing down on your head
when you've left no dry ground
to retreat to, no sanctuary
to call your own.
Tell more lies, I say,
of the half-moon kind,
and make more appointments
with your hungry, space-loving self.

Maya Shaw Gale[clxxxii]

Self-Study Practice: Self-care

1. Take a moment to self-reflect on how and when you experience misusing power toward yourself. Identify two specific examples of this.

2. The savoring and serving ideas from #3 have rich possibilities for exploration. How and when do you move between these two. What is your experience of the extremes? What is your personal tendency? Try on an emotional and physical felt sense of both savoring and serving. Imagining being with a client, notice what your experience is when you orient toward savoring, toward self, toward serving, toward saving.

3. Living good self-care is a significant right use of professional power. Reflect on your personal care and life-style habits. Using the self-assessment chart earlier in this chapter, take some time to discern which areas of self-care you do well on and which you would like to increase your skillfulness in. Pick one or two to improve. Acknowledge yourself for the ones you already do well.

4. Identify several beliefs you carry that interfere with your self-care. Next create a new belief that would serve you better. With a partner or by yourself, say or think about this new belief and notice what your experience is. This new belief may feel nourishing. If so, try living into this belief and notice what's different in your life experience with this new belief. This new belief may bring up concerns or objections in your body and/or mind. If this happens, take some time to explore what might be needed to calm these concerns so that you can stop interfering with your self-care desires and efforts. Then try living into this new belief in your imagination.

5. Go deeper in the power spiral. Take yourself around the power spiral. Notice in which direction you are best at self-care. Identify in which direction you are most challenged. What can you do to strengthen what you do well? What can you do to be better at self-care in the direction you find most challenging?

East
• clarify and refine how you receive and use guidance
South
• delve into more self-awareness
West
• practice staying connected and non-defensive
North
• get more grounded in your wisdom and skill

Influence, Values, Diversity

Story: At conclusion of an interview for couple's counseling, the wife asked the social worker for his honest assessment of their relationship (a 35 year marriage). The wife reported that the social worker said, "I always look very hard for a ray of hope for each relationship, but frankly I don't see any here. I think you should think about getting divorced. I can also refer you to another therapist." The couple were devastated and shocked and left the appointment feeling that if someone with this much education in relationship issues thought it was hopeless, it would be unlikely that they could find professional help. The social worker may have been honest, but he wasn't taking into account the amount of influence that his assessment would have and the amount of harm that his words could cause. This was an unreasonably strong judgment for an initial interview. Equally honest, and a more effective use of his power, would have been to tell the couple that considering the issues they were dealing with, he felt it would be better for them to work with another social worker.

When asked about instances when they noticed having a stronger influence than they expected, a social worker[clxxxiii] responded: *"I am generally surprised when, long after the conclusion of therapy or many years after a talk, my clients and listeners in audiences tell me how their lives were changed for the better when I had been aware of nothing extraordinary at all. I have been in disagreements with clients and not realized that the basis of the conflict may be related to the power differential, and so I have been caught off-guard, not having tracked the power of my influence."*

Influence in a up-power role can promote well-being, or be misleading, forceful, or self-serving. Exerting "undue influence" is the term used to describe misused influence. Because of the power differential, you will automatically and immediately have increased influence on your clients. Anything you say or do may have a much stronger impact than in ordinary interactions. Having influence is a part of your role and much of your success depends upon the right use of this increased influence.

Power is the potential to bring change. Influence is how we interact with our clients to bring change. There is no way to avoid having increased influence and no way to be conscious of all the influence you have.

You can, however,

- Understand more of your beliefs about power
- Increase your awareness of and sensitivity to your influence
- Do your best to use this influence in service to your clients.

Aspects of increased influence

Increased influence has a number of dimensions.

1. the stronger impact of whatever you say or do that the power differential creates
2. the subtle and overt influences of simple things like your age, sex, marital status, or race that effect interactions
3. the influence on your clients of your modeling of your values, attitudes, and style of relating
4. your core values and how you translate these into behavior
5. the diversity of explicit and implicit beliefs and behaviors around power that are attached to class, religion or philosophy, body shape and size, sexual preference, ethnic background, sex, disabilities, age, economic strata, nationality, and particular life experiences
6. what you select to focus on with your clients
7. the professional modality you use

Wise use of influence

Influence can be used appropriately in:

- promoting independence, competence, and self-confidence
- taking responsibility for your own errors
- avoiding dual relationships which are exploitative
- tracking for and resolving difficulties within the relationship
- helping clients make good choices
- modeling and teaching empowering, respectful, and skillful uses of power

Advice or direction can be offered appropriately:

- in response to a genuine and appropriate request
- in emergency or danger
- when clear or firm boundaries are needed

Self-disclosure can be used appropriately:
• to promote the therapeutic (not a personal) relationship
• to illustrate a point
• to model effective behavior
• to demonstrate and normalize vulnerability
• to show humanness

Values

In all that we do, deliberately and subtly, we influence clients with our values. Even when we focus on supporting a client's different values, our own values will be present and may influence. It is better to exert this influence in a conscious and educated way.

Any modality we use is based on ***fundamental beliefs*** about such things as:
• how change happens
• the nature of health
• causes of ill health
• the nature of good and evil
• the meaning of life
• how people should be treated
• how to respond to resistance
• how directive to be

The following qualities and abilities from Jensen and Bergin are commonly known as basic human values and goals that define well-being.[clxxxiv]

1) developing effective strategies for coping with stress
2) developing the ability to give and receive affection
3) increasing one's ability to be sensitive to feelings of others
4) becoming able to practice self-control
5) having a sense of purpose for living
6) being open, honest, and genuine
7) finding satisfaction in one's work
8) having a sense of identity and self-worth
9) being skilled in interpersonal relationships
10) being committed in marriage, family, and other relationships
11) having deepened self-awareness and motivation for growth
12) practicing good habits of physical health
13) having the capacity to experience and express compassion

"The work of the Institute for Global Ethics suggests that there are core global values that transcend individual cultures." In 1994, Rushworth Kidder[clxxxv] interviewed 24 'moral exemplars' from 16 countries. Each interview began with a common question: *"If you could create a global code of ethics, what moral values would be on it?"* They found, to their wonderment, that similar values emerge when interviewing managers around the world for a global U.S. financial services firm, participants in their ethics workshops, and groups of 8th graders. They found that for most people the concept of being ethical is synonymous with being trustworthy and having integrity.

Global attributes

The attributes of integrity and trustworthiness are:

- love
- truthfulness
- fairness
- freedom
- unity
- tolerance
- responsibility
- respect

"These responses have since been confirmed in a proprietary survey we (the IGE) conducted for the top 1,100 managers in a major U.S. financial services firm that is increasingly global in its markets. There the top values were honesty, responsibility, respect, and fairness—values that did not vary by location around the world."

Although there is much agreement about universal core values, beliefs about the right behavioral translation of these values varies across religions, political systems, and cultures. While all may agree on the value of tolerance, tolerance may not extend to those who threaten or appear to threaten harm. While all may agree about the value of freedom, this may not extend to those who have a different life-style. Fundamental values are universal; behavioral translations of these are often divergent. Divergent translations are often related to how leaders perceive differences. When differences are perceived as proof of separateness, those who are different tend to be seen and experienced as threatening and wrong, and thus excluded and de-valued, or in the extreme, terrorized. When differences are seen as aspects of "we are all one," those who are different tend to be seen and experienced as equally deserving of being treated with interest, respect, dignity and kindness. Similarities connect and differences enrich.

There are rare occasions when value differences between you and a client might be so conflicting that you would need to refer your client to someone else. These are some factors to consider.

1) You feel extreme disapproval or discomfort with your client's values.

2) You are unable to be empathic or objective.

3) You have strong concerns about the possibility that you might be imposing your values rather than inviting your client to consider another value in the context of their life and community.

Diversity

"Our differences define us, but our common humanity can redeem us. We just have to open our hearts."—Karen Armstrong[clxxxvi]

"While I, as a middle class white American, can have a small taste of the experience of oppression, I cannot begin to understand those people who have suffered with it for centuries. Most of my students in Right Use of Power classes have been white. When people of color enter the class, their withdrawal is noticeable. When we talk about power issues, they withdraw further. I have to be willing to recognize that those who have been oppressed will know much more about me than I want to realize. They have a radar that I have not had to develop nearly as well. I also recognize my own discomfort when I allow myself to go to the edge of my culture and allow space for another."

—Patti Tiberi, Right Use of Power Teacher[clxxxvii]

Following are some areas in which to be particularly attentive to possible cultural differences. This attentiveness will pay off in improved communication when you:

1)   recognize a cultural difference

2)   adapt your behavior to accommodate the difference and/or call attention to the difference to explain confusion in communication

This set of questions below by Bennett[clxxxviii] is a well-written guide to increasing your sensitivity to cultural diversity. As you see, there are many areas of cultural difference that, without being sensitized, would be difficult to be aware of. Difficulties, confusion, and distrust can easily develop out of simple lack of awareness of possible areas of difference.

Language Use
1. **Honorifics**: What are appropriate titles? When are first names appropriate (if ever)? What difference does status make in using titles?
2. **Vocabulary**: What jargon is shared by the other person (if any)? When are you using slang or culture-specific metaphors (such as football parallels or references to television shows)? What words and ideas are specific to your particular department or function?
3. **Grammar**: Are you speaking at the same level of complexity as your partner? Are you being logical or contextual in the presentation of ideas?

Communication Style
1. **Greeting Rituals:** How long is an appropriate greeting? Are compliments appropriate? Are different status people greeted differently? What physical behavior (e.g. handshaking, other touching (if any) is expected?
2. **Circular or Linear Conversation**: Are you expected to come directly to the point or should you provide more "background" information first? How will your partner react to direct approaches?
3. **Subtlety or Directness**: Should problems be confronted directly and openly or is subtle allusion and hinting more appropriate? Should compliments be given openly?

Non-Verbal Behavior
1. **Paralanguage**: How might cultural differences in "tone of voice" be affecting your perception of the other person? To what extent are you depending on tone of voice to convey feelings to someone who might not know how to interpret the tone?
2. **Body Language**: How is more pronounced gesturing or more restrained gesturing affecting your perception? How is eye contact different? Are you assuming that less eye contact means inattentiveness? What is an appropriate distance to stand or sit from the other person? When is it all right to touch the other person (if ever)?
3. **Time Language**: What is being on time? Are there cultural differences in what might be an appropriate reason to be late?

Values

1. **Individualism or Group Orientation**: How important is individual effort? When is it appropriate to get help? From whom should one receive help? How important is individual competition relative to group cooperation?
2. **Egalitarianism or Recognition of Status**: Should everyone ideally be treated the same or should people be treated differently depending on their status or relationship with you? Are you reacting negatively to what you see as "hypocrisy"?
3. **Problem solving or Acceptance**: Are troublesome situations challenges to be overcome or are they simply the way things are? Whose responsibility is problem solving?
4. **Getting Ahead or Getting Along**: Should you try to be better than your peers? When is achievement more important than affiliation (if ever)?

One of my students[clxxxix] touchingly describes her experience of being a Japanese foreign student in an American psychotherapy training program. Hiromi told me that one of the members of her class, not intending to hurt her, said, *"Your words don't have power, right? Because you don't speak English so much."* She was surprised but realized that this was exactly why she was afraid of speaking up. *"My words do not have as much power because I speak English as a second language. People will often discount me at first unless people are culturally open. And so, I feel some invisible pressure internally and from the group to be more submissive and own less power. I don't know if people mean for me to have less power."*

She told me about several other cultural differences that have been challenging to her in her participation in the program. *"In Japanese language we tend to refrain from using 'I statements' to avoid individuation. We also tend to be less direct. The personal space seems bigger in American culture compared to that of Japanese culture. I try to show the respect to teachers by referring to them as teachers, being more polite, and having more distance. In American culture it seems openness and casualness are important. In Japan, what is most important is to show appreciation through gifts so I always bring gifts."* Notice how knowing these few simple cultural differences would facilitate a safer and more productive helping relationship. Bringing gifts, keeping a respectful distance, reticence to speak about herself, take up much space, demonstrate personal power, or offer critical feedback could be understood and held within its cultural context by sensitive and aware therapists or caregivers.

In summary, this short section on diversity, honestly, is quite inadequate for attending to a multitude of serious concerns and needs, always important but even more present and significant in our increasingly diverse and increasingly interdependent world.

Story: A personal experience in an outback station in Aboriginal land in Australia speaks to power misuse and healing between two very diverse races and cultures: white and aboriginal. *We dozen "white fellas" had received the personal invitation needed to enter Aboriginal land to visit for 10 days. We had driven several thousand miles inland to the river border. On one side of the river, motor boats with ice chests of food and technical fishing equipment, on the other side barefoot aboriginal children fishing with hand held fishing lines wading at the river bank. From the river, we had driven for several days on a rutted, powder-dusted, single-lane road to get to our camp. We had been fishing, we had learned about Tea Tree medicine, we had hunted for bush food, and we had made click sticks. We knew it was a privilege to be there.*

For some of us, it had been our third visit. We had been invited to witness ceremonial dances on the first two visits. This time we were invited to join the dance. We ochered our skin with lines of white outlining our bones. We did our best to learn the dance steps. We discovered that dancing involved not just learning the steps but expanding our field of perception so that we were literally "danced" by our entrainment with the other dancers. We had felt the excitement and energy build as the lights and sounds of the truck entered the ceremonial ground. The truck bringing the boys seemed like a real living being. The boys' bodies had been elaborately painted with ancestral stories over several days of teachings by their uncles in a sacred and secret enclave. These boys stood tall and proud, receiving the admiration of the entire community as they stepped into this ceremony of boys-becoming-men. We had watched the men accept these boys and the women wail over the loss of their boy children who would no longer be allowed to speak directly to their mothers.

The three-day dance had ended in the wee hours of the morning and we had all returned to our sleeping bag "swags" for much needed sleep. The energy was high and sleep had been difficult for most of us. My experience of the night had been quite strange, especially for one who has little access to liminal information. I awoke in darkness to a feeling of being watched. I turned my head and saw what seemed like an aboriginal boy on his knees looking at me. Knowing this wasn't a real person, but truly seeing something, I made up that there was a little bush next to my swag. Others came in for breakfast with their own similar stories. Our guide, James, had been up all night feeling as if a circus had been let out.

As we packed up that day, we got word that Rex, the Head Man, and Cookie, another elder, wanted to come talk with us. This was highly unusual behavior. No one from the community except our guide Audrey had come to our camp during our visit. We had gone to their camp instead. We told them we would be honored. They arrived with a painting of a sugar bag ant colony painted by another elder, Charlie. What ensued was a most remarkable conversation that gathered its meaning as it unfolded through our interactions energetically, through gestures and expressions, and through words these elders knew in English and the words our guide knew in their language. This is the best sense we could make of it. These elders had also felt some unusual unleashed energy during the night and were trying to understand it. They seemed to feel that there was some connection between their inviting us to dance with them and this strange energy. They were concerned. They brought out the painting to show us. They told us about someone had tried to copy this painting and done it imperfectly. Soon after he had died. They spoke of stories and pointed to our notebooks and journals. They repeated over and over, "You lawmen now. You lawmen now." We began to understand that they had let us in on a level of experience and understanding that is beyond what they were used to sharing in their rare contacts with white people. They were now worried about how we would use what we had experienced. They wanted us to know that it was of enormous importance to them that we tell the truth about our experience and not make things up or be inaccurate. If we did, like the man who miscopied the painting, our lives would be in danger.

They began to talk about the "spirits" that were "loose" the night before. They didn't seem to understand what this meant and wanted to know if we had experienced this energy as well. Assured that we did, they began pointing to each of us, saying, "You good dancer! You good dancer." They then began to enact, as if on a stage, a horrific memory of an event that had happened at this station some 60 years ago. These two old men, as young boys, had hidden behind some trees in the bush and watched as bounty hunters had come and massacred their relatives. Pointing on his body to various places as if bullet holes, Rex cried, "Shoot 'em here and shoot 'em here, and here and here. Why you kill us? Why you kill us? Why you kill us?" We sat, listening, weeping. The Christian missionaries had saved the lives of many of the children by taking them away to mission schools where they were then robbed of their aboriginal lives and heritage by being given new names and taught English and

Christian ways. A number of the women in this outpost had spent years in mission schools. Rex and Cookie and a handful of others had not been found by the bounty hunters and had stayed on the land.

"You good dancers. You dance with us. You good dancers." We then began to understand that Rex and Cookie were thinking that the spirits of those who had been shot long ago had been "freed" by our willingness and interest in learning their dance and their culture. Perhaps what I had "seen" next to me in the night was a spirit now freed to be curious. It was not enough, but it seemed that we had begun to redeem the past by embracing their culture rather than taking it away. We were different. We had used our power to understand and honor their culture.

Status Power and Racism

Status (also referred to as rank) could be defined as the increased, yet unearned or partly earned (as in education and wealth) personal power that is culturally conferred and, in many cases, culturally variable. For example, in America, greater status power is given to those who are any of the following--men, white, rich, able-bodied, American citizen, Christian, well-educated, heterosexual. In America, lower status power is held by those who are, for example, poor, non-white, non-citizen, immigrant, disabled, mentally challenged, Muslim, homosexual. Obviously the more of the higher status categories you fit, the more status power you have. This status power can be used to justify hatred, violence, oppression and discrimination. And, like role power, it can also be used to heal wounds and create more actual equality. This is a daunting and humbling challenge.

Diversity and status have a complex relationship that often changes by geography and cultural context. People holding lower status are persistently discriminated against, disrespected, maligned, shamed, oppressed, exploited and physically and emotionally harmed. Some lower status categories bring deeply-rooted hateful and violent discrimination-- for example, black, native American, homosexual, and Muslim. In American society in which the gap between rich and poor and white and non-white and highly educated and non-degreed is growing, what is called white privilege is a factor that needs major and massive corrective attention.

Addressing racism--discrimination simply by virtue of racial background--is an issue of power and status that is beyond the scope of this book. Although racism has a status component, to understand racism as simply a status issue is insulting and demeaning. Racism is social and systemic injustice writ large. The few paragraphs here can serve only to shine a tiny light in this very large room. I bow to those who understand more and who are working for justice and freedom.

Changing systems of oppression and violence begins with recognizing and understanding these systems. I write these paragraphs for those of you reading this book who are, like me, steeped in the privileges of being white and highly educated. Historically, America's wealth was built on black slave labor. American democracy was written by white European men. This foundation of white men with power and slaves and Native Americans and women without power, meant, in fact, that the words, "with liberty and justice for all," applied initially to white men. Privilege itself is based on inheritance of wealth, education, empowerment, land ownership and real estate that precedes our present social circumstances. What is called white privilege, now referring to both white men and white women, is the systemic result.

The negative impacts of white privilege are beginning to be taught in many public schools starting in elementary school. Kyle Spencer[cxc] says, "*Today 'white privilege' studies center on the systemic nature of racism as well as the way it exposes minorities to daily moments of stress and unpleasantness--sometimes referred to as 'micro-aggressions.' Freedom from such worries is a privilege in and of itself, the theory goes, one that many white people are not even aware they have.*" Through these studies, white students are stepping out of a dream and realizing that the lower status people they know are living in a more challenging and dangerous world than they will ever face. [cxci]

Personally, when I am a teacher, I am well aware that I am wearing a scarf symbolic of my add-on role power. This scarf is visible to me. I also wear other symbolic greater status scarves that are visible to those of lower status but carry privileges that are invisible to me: white status, elder status, educated status, American status, able-bodied status, etc. The unearned privileges that I have taken for granted are sobering. Peggy McIntosh,[cxcii] back in 1989, identified some of the daily effects of white privilege in her life. She noted things like: "*I can, if I wish, arrange to be in the company of people of my race most of the time.*" "*I can turn on the television or open to the front page of the paper and see people of my race widely represented.*" "*When I am told about our national heritage or about 'civilization,' I am shown that people of my color made it what it is.*" "*I can arrange to protect my children most of the time from people who might not like them.*" "*I can be sure that if I need legal or medical help, my race will not work against me.*" "*I can criticize our government and talk about how much I fear its policies and behavior without being seen as a cultural outsider."* She named 26 of these advantages.

Our educational system teaches us that in democratic America "all are created equal and have equal access to life, liberty and the pursuit of happiness." History books give scant attention to the injustice, violence, and harm white people and white laws have caused Native Americans, Black Americans, and Japanese Americans to name the groups that have born the greatest abuses of power. Non-white-privileged people don't experience and assume equality and justice. White-privileged people experience and assume equal access. Their higher status privileges are taken for granted as social opportunities and treatment that everyone already has. Responses like "I don't see color," or "I'm not racist," interfere with their ability to see and own their many white privileges. At a deeper level, there is an unacknowledged psychological shadow that white people carry this is emotional rather than social and systemic. It is a cultural heritage dating to the psychological wound of slavery. When in the presence of Blacks, most white people respond with fear, a sense of "otherness," and/or shame about how their ancestors (and some of their contemporaries) treated Blacks.[cxciii]

But then, what would right use of status power and influence be? How can those who have unearned privileges use their status wisely and compassionately? Becoming informed intellectually and emotionally, personally and systemically about white privilege in relation to racism, and higher status in relation to minorities, -isms, and other lower status categories comes first.

To summarize:
> • Cultivate places where you yourself have lower rank. This will increase your sensitivity and empathy and remind you that there are highs and lows to both higher and lower rank. Learn to consciously move between up-power and down-power.[cxciv]
> • Understand and own your elevated status and the conscious and unconscious harm that unearned privilege causes.
> • Feel the pain and grief, even horror, of being part of a system that has caused, and continues to cause harm to minorities; accept that although you may not have consciously caused harm, you are part of a system that does.
> • Examine and mediate your own shadow tendencies. For example: lack of empathy, simplistic thinking, blaming the other, objectifying, creating social distance, retreating into shame, denial of differences, hopelessness, and helplessness.

• Divest white privilege from an identity of "better than," or "same as." Don't fault those with lower status for their lack of access and opportunity. Advantage leads to more advantage and disadvantage leads to more disadvantage.

• Feel your empathy, connection, and concern. Be guided by your moral compass.

• Take individual compassionate action. Speak about what you are doing to bring about change.

• Join with and accompany those who are discriminated against to work to change underlying systems.

Self-Study Practices:

1. Cultural Messages

This questionnaire is designed to help you identify the wide range of cultural messages about power and then explore how these messages have influenced you in their relationship with and use of power.

Please engage your curiosity about uncovering a few of your beliefs about power that may have been influenced by acculturated factors. These beliefs are most often subconscious. The act of bringing them to consciousness will help you understand and then use your influence more skillfully.

Self-Study practices (contributed by Patti Tiberi[cxcv]):

First, recall and share or write notes about one experience when you have been surprised by the impact of your age, sex, marital status, race, or nationality.

What is the impact of your sex, race, ethnic background, education, financial status, nationality, marital status, body size and/or shape, religious preference, class, age, sexual orientation, disabilities, military experience, English as second language, status as an immigrant, extended family, primary decision-maker/head of household, involvement in groups or clubs.....? *Choose several of these factors that seem particularly interesting, charged, or relevant.*

Two questions that go with each category are:
1. What messages about power have you received in relation to this factor?
2. In what way do these messages show up in how you use your power with your clients?

(One person's example: 1. "I received the message that women should stay in the background and support men, so 2. I'm reluctant to take charge or be directive with my clients.")

Two questions that can be asked about the information gathered from the above.
1. In what ways have these messages or beliefs caused you to feel disempowered?
2. What are some new ways you thinking, feeling, or acting that would allow you to feel more empowered or would mediate any negative impact of your acculturated beliefs?

(One person's example: 1. "Well, it's disempowering, for obvious reasons, but also empowering because I have learned to value the power of being receptive. 2. I am teaching myself to be more assertive and to have some 'chutzpa.'")

2. Of Local Interest

Get curious and find out about the influence that you have with your family, friends, and support system. (This is an opportunity that is not so freely and open-endedly available when you are with your clients.) Use this information to deepen your sensitivity to the increased influence that you also have with your clients. Let it help you examine unconscious impacts.

3. Top 10 Values

List your top 10 values. Explore how you react when a client or colleague doesn't agree with one of them. Reflect on how you react when a client or colleague agrees with a value and then does not act or speak in accordance with this value.

Leadership & Power Dynamics

"Power is not something we should (or can) avoid, nor is it something that necessarily involves domination and submission. We are negotiating power every waking instant of our social lives...When we see equality, we are seeking an effective balance of power, not the absence of power. We use it to win consent and social cohesion, not just compliance. To be human is to be immersed in power dynamics."[cxcvi]

"I feel like I'm now growing up in my profession," said a student. "No longer am I just a movement therapist who wants to help people. I am a leader. I am becoming a model for how to use power wisely, consciously, and with skill. I understand that it's not enough to just be a good person and have good intentions. I must be myself in my own powerful way that does more than not do harm, but rather stays in right relationship and repairs harm and teaches others how to use power benevolently."[cxcvii]

Uses of power that promote sustainable and experiential well-being and abuses of power that cause harm are most impactful from leadership positions. Leadership is too complex a topic to cover in any depth in a few pages, but here are several ideas that fit intrinsically with the Right Use of Power approach.

Leadership styles and their dynamics

Four kinds of leadership and use of power are connected to the four power spiral dimensions. As you go through these, you will likely discover that there are one or two leadership styles with which you feel most comfortable.   You may also notice that the **best leaders pull from all four of the power styles** although they have one or two that are most native to them.   You might also find that you lead a bit more from one style or another in different life contexts, like when you are with peers or family compared to when you are in an up-power role.

Acknowledge and strengthen these leadership styles in your professional and personal life. Choose one leadership style in which you would like to become more skilled. Find ways to increase your facility in this area. Since it is not reasonable to expect to do every style well, it is helpful to accept and accommodate for your less competent styles.

Leadership Styles/Power Styles

•
• *Leading from information*
Brilliance: projecting the power of ideas and organization. Is well-organized, clear and-detail-oriented; is well-prepared and presents well; responds concisely to questions; is intellectually inspiring and engaging; assesses people and progress by details, clarity, and understanding; and provides for safety and trust through good boundaries and clarity.
Examples: Barbara Marx Hubbard, Albert Einstein, Stephen Hawking, Angela Merkel, Ken Wilber
Wilber quadrant: It *(outside the individual)*
Up-power role challenge: unprepared to hold increased power
Shadow: Can be dry and overwhelm with information and details; can be out of touch with feelings and impatient with the maintenance aspect of leadership; can use information to mislead or manipulate.
Direction: East

•
• *Leading from Self*
Brilliance: projecting the power of presence and vitality. Is lively and engaging; uses his or her personality to draw people in; is warm and genial; shares personal stories, jokes, insights; is charismatic, charming, magnetic and dynamic; tracks for and assesses aliveness and commitment; inspires trust and safety through strength and persuasiveness.
Examples: Archbishop Desmond Tutu, Oprah Winfrey, Billy Graham, Tony Robbins, Elizabeth Warren
Wilber quadrant: I *(inside the individual)*
Up-power role challenge: ego over-identification with increased power
Shadow: Can get caught up in their ego and over-identify with their up-power role; can prioritize their own needs and desires; can have great difficulty receiving constructive feedback, giving credit to others and being in a down-power position to anyone else.
Direction: South

•
• *Leading from Connectedness*
Brilliance: projecting the power of support and connectedness.
Is relationally skilled and good at communication; is appreciative, warm, inclusive, interactive and receptive; understands systems; encourages active participation; cares about justice and fairness; tracks and assesses for healthy, sustaining connections; creates trust and safety through interpersonal interactions.
Examples: Mr. Rogers, Jim Sinegal (CEO of Costco), Dalai Lama, Margaret Mead, Mother Theresa
Wilber quadrant: We *(the inside of the collective)*
Up-power role challenge: reluctance to own increased power and responsibility
Shadow: Can get so lost in relationship dynamics and loyalties that the task takes a back seat; can under-use or abandon up-power role; can lose direction; can create chaos and confusion
Direction: West

•
• *Leading from Vision*
Brilliance: projecting the power of the possible and the whole.
Sees larger perspectives; is integrative, creative, idealistic and inspiring; is flexible and spontaneous; is an out-of-the-box visionary. Tracks and assesses for commitment to the cause and creates trust and safety through the goodness of the vision.
Examples: Mahatma Gandhi, Jean Houston, Al Gore, Steve Jobs, Martin Luther King
Wilber quadrant: Its *(the outside of the collective)*
Up-power role challenge: disassociation from impact
Shadow: Can become lost in their vision and not be able to see for themselves or help their followers do the practical tasks of getting to the vision; can get ungrounded and lose connection; can lose momentum and support by promising more than is reasonable and moving too far ahead of their followers.
Direction: North

North—leading from Vision

West—Leading from Connectedness   Leadership from 4 directions   East—leading from information

South—Leading from Self

Five Values of Effective Leadership

Mark Gerzon [cxcviii] is an international mediator who has worked with corporate leaders, public officials and civic groups throughout the world to foster constructive, collaborative approaches to global issues. In his book, *Leading Beyond Borders*, Mark describes five values of effective and skillful leadership that work beyond borders rather than behind borders. **These values are the essence of Right Use of Power.** Guided by these values, helping professionals can earn and increase trust in their leadership and learn to work systemically on behalf of the whole.

Integrity: This is the ability to witness the whole and to use systems thinking. Integrity involves grasping as many dimensions as possible and the deep self-awareness of knowing oneself, including shadow. It requires being humble and willful, decisive and reflective, and solitary and collaborative.

Learning: The value of learning leads to focusing on inquiry—strategic questioning that leads to answers beyond the borders of one's thinking; listening—engaging with new information that challenges one's assumptions; and witnessing—seeing self and other fully and accurately.

Trust: For trust to flourish, it must grow naturally in soil that is rich in integrity. It includes sincerity—the intention to keep one's word, competence—the skill and capacity to keep commitments, and reliability developing a track record of accountability. Building trust requires a safe container, conscious communication, and dialogue.

Bridging: This is a specific process of analysis—thinking through issues and identifying stakeholders, convening—the art of bringing stakeholders together, and collaboration—willingness and capacity to engage in co-operative actions.

Synergy: The goal is to create a whole that is more than the sum of its parts. This new whole should be innovative in that it adds value; just in that value is shared; and sustainable in that value endures.

Most Important Leadership Qualities and Skills

Before moving into some information about power dynamics, here is a list of the best leadership qualities as researched by Dacher Keltner.[cxcix]

- reconciling conflict
- negotiating
- fairness and respect
- smoothing over tensions
- enforcing group norms
- co-operation
- humility

To these I would add several things that are implied: social engagement skills, compassion, and the ability to self-reflect and self-correct.

Power Dynamics

"The moving forces of any kind, or the laws relating to them," [cc] is the definition of dynamics. There are many engaging and challenging dynamics inherent to power positions. Understanding and working with these is an on-going process well worth your effort and attention. Your effectiveness and satisfaction as a leader depends on your understanding and personal work with these issues. This is an area of self study of the impact of your use of power and the subtleties of power dynamics. In the context of naming power dynamics, the following is a summary of some themes that have been mentioned in other chapters of this book:

1. Context of the Therapeutic Relationship:

The therapeutic relationship is consciously set up to be an ideal and time-limited one. This context can facilitate powerful healing, but it is also a distortion of what is possible in normal, everyday relationships. Clients can develop unrealistic expectations and/or dysfunctional dependencies.

Therapists can develop an unrealistic sense of effectiveness and an attachment to the kind of emotional closeness that they participate in through being in service to another that is by design not reciprocal.

2. Seduction of Adulation:

Therapists, leaders, teachers get both adulated and hated. It is *very* easy to lose perspective in either extreme. Both admiration and criticism are distortions that come with the role. It is especially easy to take refuge in and/or be seduced by adulation, which inhibits learning and self-correcting. One teacher received some written feedback that he had "fallen asleep and was teaching the material in a tired way." This helped him revive his curriculum.

3. Transpersonal Love:

Respect, appreciation, and transpersonal love from a student to a teacher or therapist is a valuable component for healing and learning. However, it can be very easy to confuse this transpersonal love with romantic love, for either or both teacher and student. Some of the qualities may feel the same between the two forms of love, but the distortion created by the power differential and role differences make it extremely important and challenging to recognize the difference between the two and to act from this difference.

4. Lifetime Role:

Therapists who have been in the profession for 10, 20, 30 years may become so embedded in their therapist persona (boundaries, being of service, sexuality, putting personal needs and desires aside, attentive and reflective listening style, etc.) that they find it difficult to shift out of role appropriately in other life arenas. One therapist who was single found herself continually meeting potential romantic partners who found themselves drawn to her just as a friend. She was so used to her therapist persona that she had a difficult time bringing her attraction and sexuality forward in appropriate social situations. Therapeutic skill can, in fact, be one of the most sophisticated of defense mechanisms.

5) Down-power:

A person in a position of less power has a tendency to feel and act victimized. Feeling or being shamed can exaggerate this tendency. The Down-power person in the power differential may get into a "tunnel" of proving their worth; or on the other hand, de-compensate and begin acting helpless. Both parties may collude in a self-generating and self-fulfilling system. When the Down-power person doesn't stand up for him/her self the up-power person begins to disrespect the Down-power person who then de-compensates even more, and so on.

6) Feedback Loop:

Leaders often fail to understand the interruption of the normal feedback loop that happens when there is a power differential (namely that those lower in the power hierarchy have an investment in being liked, included, and valued and thus will tend to tell those higher up only, or primarily, positive things). Leaders therefore, become more and more confident about their perceptions and less and less aware that they are not getting the full or accurate picture no matter how carefully they listen to the feedback that comes to them. The leader then gets more and more out of touch and continues to make the same mistakes.

7) Diversity:

"Maturity is the ability to differentiate and then integrate the differences in the apparently similar and the similarities in the apparently different." —Yvonne Agazarian[cci]

Will Schutz[ccii] has identified some stages of group development that are: **inclusion** (bonding around similarities), **control** (chaos and power issues—identification of differences, polarizing differences, bonding around differences), and **affection** (intimacy that comes from learning not only to tolerate, but to value differences).

Sub-groups tend to polarize around differences including differences in the use of power. In working with differences, the goal is to respect and use differences for the greatest good. This learning generally has three stages: experiencing and naming differences; bonding around similarities and tolerating differences; and then honoring, valuing, and relying on differences.

8) Bonding:

The bond between the one who is judging and the one who is judged is extremely compelling and primary. We all need to feel "good enough" and we will continue to obsess about knocking on the door of the one important person who is critical or who has power over us even when we experience being "enough" elsewhere in our lives. The compelling power in this relationship exists on both sides. The judger is equally linked with the judged through their need to be better than or their need for control.

9) Scapegoating:

Scapegoating can happen through the "scapegoat" either taking or being given too much responsibility for things that aren't working. People may be scapegoated for a wide variety of reasons, from their inability to act on their own behalf, to their need to avoid conflict, to their lack of self-esteem, to their devotion to service, to the naive hope that if they take some responsibility, others will take their share.

10) As Above:

"As above, so below." In power dynamics, the strengths and the limitations of those in positions of authority tend to pervade the atmosphere of the whole organization. If the leader(s) don't acknowledge the followers, the followers are unlikely to acknowledge each other.

11) Modeling:

There is an interesting phenomenon called, "moral elevation." This is described as "an emotional state that leads us to act virtuously when exposed to the virtue of others. In experiments, participants who are brought face to face with others' gratitude or giving behavior are more likely to display those virtues themselves."[cciii] As a leader, living by and putting your values into action will, without even talking about it, positively effect those you are leading.

11) Perspective:

"The fish are the last to discover water." The things that may be so obvious to others outside the system are the hardest to see within the system.

12) Respect:

Acknowledgment, Appreciation, and Respect may be the three most important things for leaders to remember to offer.

13) Requests for Change:

Power relations will be more effective and satisfying the more you develop skill in making complaints with a request for change that is specific and behavioral. Character comments such as "You always . . ." and vague requests such as "be more responsible" aren't helpful.

14) Pay it Forward:

Uses of power to repair harm and promote well-being, even when skillful, aren't always met with appreciation and respect and don't always turn out as intended. There is an intrinsic satisfaction, value, and impact in doing the right thing, even when the positive or healing result is not readily apparent. Goodness often pays itself forward.

These notes are theories gathered from my personal experience and are included here to provoke thought and discussion and to convey the wide range of conscious and unconscious systems that are involved in power dynamics. These theories are not all-inclusive and may or may not align with your own experience. In addition, they may be applied to larger circles than those of health care professionals. In all humility, I offer these theories as pieces of a platform upon which much needs to be built.

Understanding, exploring, and becoming more facile with leadership and power dynamics is an on-going challenge and engagement with who you are and how you impact people. In a chapter on Leadership in the book *Presence*, author Peter Senge[cciv] talks about leadership in history. *"One of the oldest ideas about leadership is that 'with power must come wisdom'—an idea that seems to date from the period when larger city states were forming in china and Greece about twenty-five hundred years ago."* *"Today,"* Betty Sue Flowers adds, *"our leaders are more likely to be technologists than philosophers, focused on gaining and using power, driving change, influencing people, and maintaining an appearance of control."* *"The old idea that those in positions [of]... influence must be committed to cultivation of moral development"* must once again become the dominant philosophy. Cultivation involves *"develop[ing] a capacity for delayed gratification, for seeing longer-term effects of actions, [and] for achieving quietness of mind."* Adds Otto Scharmer, *"the cultivated self is a leader's greatest tool."*

Balancing Hierarchy and Equality

"Leaders in complex systems cannot control the behavior of all agents in the system. They cannot control changes either inside or outside their organizations. The alternative is to engage authentically with others to learn about and respond to changes as they arise. Leaders must be as willing to be transformed as they are to transform others."—Genda Eoyang[ccv]

Moving in the direction of more humanistic and value-driven organizations and leadership styles requires a change in relationship to hierarchy (power differential). Unfortunately, hierarchy is often seen as the enemy of collaborative organizations that want to honor, respect, and empower their employees, faculty, professionals, or supervisees. Just as it is often thought that one must choose between power as strength and power as connectedness, it can seem that as a leader, one must choose between vertical control and direction and horizontal empowerment and collaboration. Leading-edge organizations understand that there is ethical and functional value in both hierarchy and collaboration. For an organization to be healthy, vibrant and co-creative, leaders must be strong, directive, and accountable as well as connected, collaborative, and respectful.

Leaders are finding that the right balance of role hierarchy and role equality is essential to creating a vibrant and healthy group. Looking at this on a continuum, too much hierarchy can result in distrust, lack of engagement, exploitation, reduced creativity, and strong push-back. Too much equality can reduce productivity, obscure accountability, impede decision-making, flatten the environment, and confuse friendship and task loyalties. Not enough of either role hierarchy or role equality results in chaos. Leadership ability to move flexibly along the continuum staying away from the unhealthy extremes is an important skill. I call this **role power fluidity.** It takes training, awareness and sensitivity to move fluidly between up-power and down-power roles.

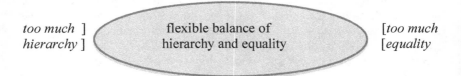

too much]   flexible balance of   [*too much*
hierarchy]   hierarchy and equality   [*equality*

Summarizing:
Value of Role Hierarchy
        Clarify responsibilities
        See the biggest picture
        Create a safe environment
        Assign and Assess
        Hold accountability
        Take charge when needed
        Make tough decisions when needed

Holding an Up-power (hierarchical) Position in a Collaborative Way--
Skills and Challenges
        Avoiding the negative effects of increased power
        Being self-aware, self-reflecting, and self-correcting
        Staying connected and resolving issues
        Being respectful, appreciative, and inclusive
        Taking charge and making tough decisions

Value of Role Equality
        Inclusion
        Co-operation
        Creativity
        Camaraderie
        Co-ownership
        Mutual empowerment

Holding a Down-power Position in a Collaborative Way--
Skills and Challenges

      Giving appreciative and constructive feedback
      Accepting tough decisions
      Avoiding helplessness and passivity
      Not expecting to be favored or treated as a friend

Using Hierarchy Collaboratively

Standing in your strength while staying in your heart requires much more skill, sensitivity and awareness than choosing just one or the other. *Story: The new Executive Director of a mental health clinic called to consult with me because she felt that the clinic was "falling apart at the seams." Teams were not holding each other accountable. The atmosphere felt somehow sloppy and lazy. People were talking behind each other's backs. Her vision for the clinic was that she would be the friendly, encouraging, supportive, behind-the-scenes leader who would help everyone work well together. We had a several hour staff meeting. In addressing how things were going, I asked everyone to place themselves in the room in relationship to each other. I watched as the ED quietly walked to the side of the room and sat down. Others stood still, others wandered around. The atmosphere felt awkward and unclear. I went to the ED and quietly asked her if she would be willing to see what happened if she stood up and walked to the center of the room. She did. Almost immediately the rest of the staff found their places. The staff needed her to say yes to her role power as ED. They needed her strength, sense of the organizational whole, her direction, decisiveness, boundaries, and ability to hold staff accountable. She already had the skill set for which she had been hired: empathy, kindness, respectfulness, creativity, positive attitude, and ability to work collaboratively with others. Adding the new skill set that came with owning the increased power of her role, gave new life to the clinic, she reported when we had a follow-up call six months later.*

Here are several challenges in which a facility with role-power fluidity can be useful.

Challenge of Discernment

The key to healthy and effective leadership is mastery of the challenge of being wise and skillful both with strength and with relationships. It is to be strong with kindness and respect, and to be connected with clear boundaries. I want to mention several particular challenges. One is the challenge of discerning when it is best to be collaborative and when it is best to make a firm and clear hierarchical decision. *Story: I interviewed a recently retired and much loved, respected and effective Chief Judge. "I know you were very collaborative. Were there any times when you needed to take charge and make top down decision?" "Well, yes, there were two times in fifteen years. I quickly learned how strong an impact my very presence had on the 160 employees who worked under me. I once wrote a quick email asking a senior management employee what he thought about an idea I had. Five minutes later he was racing up the stairs and into my office to respond--as if he thought that if he didn't respond instantly, I wouldn't like him and his job would be at risk. Yikes, I thought. Certainly, this was a different impact than my intention, which was for him to think about it for a couple weeks, or whatever, and then get back to me. It was so simple, but I really GOT it about my up-power impact.*

So back to the two times as Chief Judge that I needed to make a tough and non-negotiable decision. The first was the dress code. My predecessor did not seem to care about this, so people were wearing jeans and showing midriffs and t-shirts with funky slogans on them and flip-flops. You get the idea. I always wore a suit, silk blouse, heels. I thought about creating a committee but realized that if the committee didn't come up with a dress code that I agreed with, I couldn't live with it, and would not be able to follow their conclusions. So, I thought about it a long time and tried to make code that would be something they could live with even if they didn't like it. Like, jeans were okay and t-shirts without words, but no open midriff and no flip-flops. There were a few other things on the list. But I knew this was a decision that was not only <u>mine</u> to make but important for me to make, and it wasn't negotiable. The second time was about animals at work. Again, my predecessor had allowed animals. This was another non-negotiable for me. No animals. One of my responsibilities as Chief Judge was to see the justice center from all points of view, including the general public coming into the center. Animals simply did not give the business impression that I wanted the public to experience.

Challenge of Mixing Multiple Kinds of Relationship

The second challenge I want to mention is the challenge of being relational within a power differential context. When collaboration is a strong value, relationships naturally develop in a more personal and caring way. This is a good thing. The challenge comes when the up-power role responsibilities require the leader to make a decision based on factors bigger and more complex than the personal desires, feelings and opinions of the person in the down-power role. This can be confusing and painful. *Story: Nancy was the Trainer of an extended psychotherapy program. Because the program involved students practicing with each other, she needed a team of graduate assistants how had taken the course and were skilled in the techniques. In prior trainings, she had become personally close with several of the assistants as friends and colleagues. She knew that one of these assistants was in some emotional pain. In the present situation, Nancy announced to the class that after the break, everyone would be returning to small practice groups with their assistant. After the break, two assistants went off to do personal work with each other and didn't return to provide for their groups leaving Nancy and the other assistants to fill in for them. Nancy was angry that the assistants had put their own needs ahead of the needs of the students and not even consulted with her. The assistants thought that because of their friendship Nancy would, of course, support them in taking care of themselves. Nancy did want to support them, but her bigger responsibility was to the students who didn't get the care and support they needed and were paying for. Sadly, the situation escalated so much with anger and recriminations that the two assistants quit and the friendships were not repaired. Although their role-expectations as assistants was quite clear, they were apparently unable to shift from their friend and student roles in which personal healing and self-care is the focus, into their teaching role in which the students healing comes first.* The expectations of a friendship and the responsibilities of a role are sometimes the same and sometimes different.

Another version of this challenge shows up when those in either up- or down-power roles have difficulty distinguishing and switching between interpersonally-focused interactions and task-focused interactions. For example, a teacher may focus so much on being liked and on making sure everyone is getting along that the curriculum gets ignored. Managing the balance of task and relationship maintenance is one of the responsibilities of the up-power role. Here's another example. *Story: Mario hired Jeff for his mental health team because he felt a strong affinity with him. They worked together well. However, other members of the team began to notice that Jeff's ideas and desires got more attention and that he wasn't being held to the same level of accountability. Mario, on the up-power side, was unaware of being preferential and how this was interfering with the effective functioning of the team in their jobs. Jeff, on the down-power side, had blended personal with task and could not see that sometimes more focus on the task is required. Feedback from the rest of the team helped both of them to shift their focus appropriately.*

Down-power Influence

When we say fully own and skillfully and compassionately use the power of whatever role we are in, professional power differential relationships are at their best. We all know what it's like to be in each role. Therapist and then client, therapist and then supervisee, teacher and then student, assistant and then therapist: up-power to down-power, down-power to up-power. We can sense the difference in the feeling and responsibility of each role position. We understand the 150% principle that gives greater responsibility for the health of the relationship to the up-power person.

However, it is a human experience that not all therapists, supervisors, teachers, employers use their up-power well. Misuses of up-power abound--both minor and major. So, how can being informed about right use of up-power help you when a superior is being unskillful, insensitive, disrespectful, ineffective or worse? Use your down-power influence. This is what I call the set of awarenesses, skills, and strategies that can be used to help someone who is misusing their up-power role to shift toward more sensitive and skillful use of their power.

Here's a chart that gives an overall picture.

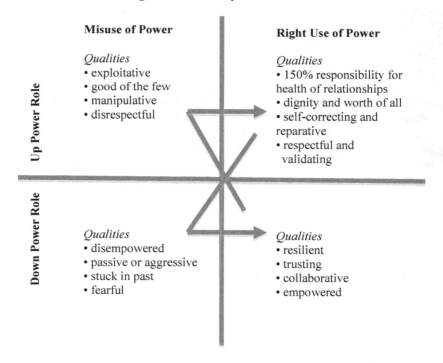

Here the chart is divided into four quadrants. Power differential relationships in which those in <u>both</u> up-power and down-power roles say "yes" to their roles are the most satisfying and functional. Sometimes, when in an up-power role, you will need to help a client or student learn how to understand and use his or her down-power role better. You will be using your upper right quadrant skills to help them move from the lower left quadrant to the lower right quadrant.

The other arrow in the chart is the place for down-power influence. This is when your superior is misusing their power and you want to use your down-power influence to help them move from the upper left quadrant to the upper right quadrant. Using down-power influence is even more challenging than wise use of up-power leadership skills. Using down-power influence requires exceptional skill, sensitivity, awareness, and flexibility. The reason it is more challenging is because you are at some risk of being hurt. You could be fired, disliked, discriminated against, humiliated, shamed, scapegoated, or blamed. You could become the "lightning rod" for a whole group or system, a most painful position. Or you could be very effective, but not get your way. Or the seeds you plant may not grow for several seasons. Story: *Jonathan was upset and discouraged about how some strong feedback he gave to the Trainer of his psychotherapy program was received. He felt blamed and ostracized and left the program. Only later did he hear how much the Trainer had learned and self-corrected with the next group. Jonathan had done the right thing but might not have gotten so hurt if he had invited others who felt the same way to join him in the complaint.*

Here's a story about working with others to make a change. *Jim's supervisor made it a practice to include the therapists he was mentoring in his groups as full participants along with the clients they were seeing in private sessions. Jim had spoken with his supervisor about his discomfort with being simultaneously both a therapist and a group member, but the supervisor did not change his approach. Jim talked with the other mentorees and found that they also found this an uncomfortable and unmanageable dual role. They decided that when all the group members were asked to pair up for a process, Jim would tell the group simply that since he felt professionally uncomfortable with this he would be role-playing in the exercise rather than being himself. The other mentorees then stated they would be too. Their plan was effective. By working together, they reduced the risk of one of them being fired. By choosing another solution, they had changed the format without shaming their supervisor.*

It is good to do the right thing, of course. But doing the right thing sensitively and skillfully is even better. So, what kind of skills and strategies are most helpful in using down-power influence? In my trainings, I ask people to pair up in up-power and down-power roles. The down-power person spends seven minutes using their best effort to resolve a problem with their up-power partner. The up-power person is instructed "not to be impossible." They were interested to see how much movement happened in just seven minutes. Almost every pair at least got back into connection with each other. Often it feels that conflict resolution is going to take forever but it doesn't have to. Debriefing with the up-power people then brings out what approaches were most helpful. Here is a list of what the up-power people most often said worked for them.

> *I felt your empathy.*
> *You actually offered a solution instead of just blaming and*
> > *complaining.*
> *You asked for a good time to talk.*
> *You listened and were respectful.*
> *You were clear and simple and had examples.*

In addition, here is a list of additional suggestions to try. Also refer to the suggestions on pages _____.

Down-Power Strategies for Working with People in Up-Power Roles

1. Offer authentic appreciations.
2. Link a complaint with a request for change.
3. Ask for a good time to talk.
4. Avoid taking something on alone when there is significant risk—join with others.
5. Be specific and describe the (negative) impact of the superior's behavior on you and/or the system.
6. Use simplicity, consistency, persistency.
7. Name possible solutions and be willing to be part of the solution.
8. Be clear about what outcome you want; then don't be attached to this particular outcome.
9. Try not to put the superior on the spot.
10. Try to understand his or her position even if you don't agree with it.
11. Focus more on how you want things to be in the future and less on the past.
12. Identify possible differences in leadership or communication style that may be causing conflict.
13. Find out where you have positive leverage and use it.

14. Stand in your strength and stay in your heart. Be forceful but also compassionate.

15. Ask your superior for feedback and respond to it.

16. When you CAN'T do what you want to do, identify what you CAN do.

17. Change a gripe into a curiosity about what might be possible.

18. Ask for a response by saying something like, "I need to know that you've heard me."

19. Learn when to persist and when to let go.

20. Try to have the largest possible perspective on the situation.

21. Enlist your superior in advocating for something or someone.

22. Plant seeds of change and then water them.

23. Be clear and direct, calm and authentic.

24. Evaluate the likely impacts of various alternative solutions.

25. Understand when you are triggered; then wait for a time when you are calmer.

26. "If you want a kitten, start by asking for a horse," i.e., use bargaining strategy.

27. Look for a WIN/WIN solution. 28. Use humor.

29. Demonstrate that you are listening to and understanding the superior.

30. Describe the likely impacts of various alternative solutions.

Be smart, creative, and compassionate. Don't disempower yourself and give up when faced with misuses of power by superiors. In our culture that is rife with misunderstandings, misuses, and abuses of power it is natural to feel hopeless and helpless to bring about change. By assuming the impossibility of change, we inadvertently collude with the dominant idea about power--that it is forceful, disrespectful, greedy, and exploitive. I use the word down-power influence instead of down-power leadership because I don't want to confuse the strategies of down-power influence with taking over the up-power role and responsibilities. Down-power influence is more about owning and influentially using the power that belongs to the down-power role.

Self-Study: Leading and Following

1. Consciousness, empathy, and skillfulness is needed in both power differential roles. Here's a checklist of a few dynamics to be conscious of when using your power in either role.

Leader/Helping Professional Power Considerations

_____ 1. Sometimes I don't take ownership of my power role.
_____ 2. Sometimes I have blurred or poor role boundaries and limits.
_____ 3. Sometimes I am arrogant or over-use my role power.
_____ 4. Sometimes I have great content, but poor timing.
_____ 5. Sometimes I have great timing, but poor content.
_____ 6. Sometimes I'm unwilling to be direct or take a stand.
_____ 7. Sometimes I'm not in good contact with my client or group.
_____ 8. Sometimes I try to use or change rules to avoid working with a relationship.
_____ 9. Sometimes I am too nice or too empathic.
_____ 10. Sometimes I don't honor or work with differences well.

Follower/Client Considerations:

_____ 1. Sometimes I hide under the leader.
_____ 2. Sometimes I engage in too much questioning and doubting.
_____ 3. Sometimes I undermine the leader.
_____ 4. Sometimes I compete with the leader.
_____ 5. Sometimes I pretend to go along.
_____ 6. Sometimes I complain without suggesting a change.
_____ 7. Sometimes I am half-present and half-hearted.
_____ 8. Sometimes I don't follow through with my agreements.
_____ 9. Sometimes I'm not emotionally available.
_____ 10. Sometimes I am not direct with my responses.

To increase your skillfulness, pick one or several of these considerations to shift.

2. What would Yoda do?

Name a personal hero. Think of a challenge and think about how this person would respond. Imagine what approach and what actions this person might make.

Challenges

Story: He was a well-loved music teacher. He loved his students. After several months of therapy, he told his therapist that he was ready to talk about something he hadn't had the trust to bring up before, and even then wasn't sure how it would be received. He had felt for a while that something about the way he loved his students, especially the boys, wasn't right. Like he had noticed that when he gave one of the boys a hug, he was grasping on, wanting to father him, wanting to give him more than a teacher should. He had then had a dream that he was holding one of his students and then in the dream the student was holding him. The therapist appreciated his courage and helped him explore what was going on. His father had died when he was six and he had experienced an aching longing for father love and attention that he felt as an adult as a deep, vacant place in his chest. In paying attention to this place in his chest, it became clear that this was the emptiness he was trying to fill when he was hugging his students. Understanding this strong need from his childhood helped him find other ways to connect and be nourished—filling himself with his music, reaching out more to friends, being more playful. His love for his students then shifted dramatically to more appropriate expression. His courage in bringing this issue to therapy resulted in pro-active behavior that prevented serious harm to his students.

Ethical pro-activity is precautionary in that by being pro-active, we put attention toward knowing ourselves and understanding our impact. It helps us consciously avoid mistakes we might be particularly prone to make due to our personal wounding, blind spots, habitual responses, naiveté, fear or shame. This stance is the Precautionary Principle applied to caregiver ethics.

The Precautionary Principle states that because of scientific uncertainty and the likelihood of harm, we must take precautionary action **before** we encounter danger rather than waiting for harm to happen. The Precautionary Principle was so-named in the 1980s and has since been used, especially in Europe, in the political and environmental realm of complex law and treaty making. The Precautionary Principle is a vital philosophy and way of living and acting in the world.[ccvi] The Precautionary

Principle couples science with ethics and bases values in actions that promote sustainable well-being.

Acting with ethical integrity and skill will always have its challenges. These challenges can be situational, cultural, and/or personal. Some of the factors that contribute to the challenges include:

- Our impact is often different than our intention.
- It's a human condition to be vulnerable to making mistakes.
- When we feel shame about misuses of power or about unresolved difficulties, we don't want them known.
- When we avoid conflict, we interrupt the impulse to resolve and repair.
- Professionals are consciously or unconsciously expected to be beyond reproach.
- Aspiration is often not acknowledged.
- Those in positions of power and trust often don't receive accurate or needed feedback. When they do receive feedback, they often respond defensively or not at all.
- Unmet personal, social, intimacy, or financial needs interfere with making clear and wise choices.
- Transference and counter-transference issues cause confusion and exaggerated responses.
- We may not know until much later that someone felt hurt.
- We may not admit or accept our limitations. Limitations are often seen as imperfections to be hidden. Awareness of limitations is good leadership and allows us to make accommodations.

Helping professionals often receive ethics training before they have had much experience with clients. A group of new counselors was asked about what most surprised or troubled them in relation to the ethical use of their power and influence. The following are their responses to the sentence:

I have been most surprised, challenged, or troubled by:

- *how often my impact does not match my intention*
- *how much subtle transference and counter-transference happens*
- *how often I think I've resolved a conflict or misunderstanding yet it reappears*

- *the variety of ways, both subtle and obvious, in which my clients give me important information about themselves and their concerns*

- *how fragile my self-confidence can be and what a wide range of responses I use—from shrinking back to trying to convince and defend*

- *How easily I want to give advice and be attached to my agenda or interpretation.*

- *how easy it is to be tempted by sexual feelings and to confuse transpersonal compassion with personal love*

Ethical pro-activity with skill and awareness is the outcome of ongoing self-exploration.

When thinking about your own habits, temptations, and defenses, I offer you another perspective. Consider the challenges faced by prisoners as they adjust to life in prison and learn to take responsibility for their behavior and impact on others. Here's a letter written by T.M. from prison. *"Martin Luther King said something like the true mark of growth isn't how a man acts when or during times of comfort and happiness, rather how he acts during times of trials and controversy. I put that to the test last week. On my way to chow the Ass't. Chief of Security pulled me aside and searched me. My shoes had a hole in the heel from daily wear. He accused me of using it as a hiding spot for contraband. He told me to go to my room and don't leave it until he came to pick them up. I didn't protest or complain. I didn't say a word the whole time. I came to my room. I sat in there until the next day. I missed breakfast, supper and my shower. When the Sgt. came to pick them up I didn't say nothing. I just handed them to her. When she asked what I wanted done with them, I said, 'Put them on the Chief's desk 'cause he wants them so bad.' That was it. That was the best behavior I ever displayed in a situation such as this. Last year I would have been writing this letter from segregation. . . . My resolve is to pray for them [the officers] every day and show them compassion even when they are adverse to me, and want to power thrust on me. I am not the same person I was. . . Anger is the cloud that obscures positive choices and clear thought processes. I have fallen victim to it countless times. . . . The normal person takes them a few precious moments to assess and evaluate the consequences of the choices he or she may have. That's why we are in prison, 'cause we did not take the time to think of our consequences. When I killed someone I wasn't thinking of Okay, what are my consequences here? Who will this effect and what kind of impact will this have?. . . . After all this time, [I still remember] I was thinking, 'I will teach this person a lesson of stealing from me. I am going to set an example for anyone who thinks of stealing from me.' I wasn't thinking normal."* [ccvii] T. M. has learned many things--to pause and think about consequences, to stay calm and not over-react, and to use down-power influence even when being mistreated. These are remarkable lessons for anyone, let alone someone in prison for murder.

Barriers

Each aspect of the Power Spiral has a particular quality of challenge or barrier. The power spiral barriers are based on the Sensitivity Cycle model from the Hakomi Method. [ccviii] In this model, increasing sensitivity, peacefulness, and effectiveness occur through moving around the Sensitivity Cycle. There are four aspects to this cycle: Clarity, Effectiveness, Satisfaction, and Relaxation. All four are necessary for success. First you become clear about what is needed. Then you take effective action. With effective action, you feel satisfied, and when satisfied you can relax, let go and get ready for the next round of the cycle. **Barriers** are habits or beliefs that interfere with your progress around the cycle. The four barriers corresponding with the four aspects are: Insight Barrier, Response Barrier, Nourishment Barrier, Completion Barrier. In the Power Spiral, the barriers that correspond with each dimension are shown in this diagram. There are also **Resources** available at each dimension. As with the Sensitivity Cycle, you may begin the cycle at any of the barriers or resources.

Being informed leads to being more aware. Increased consciousness engages compassion and leads to more connectedness and accountability. More connectedness enhances skillfulness. Greater empowerment leads into the next spiral of being more informed and so on.

To illuminate this process, here are some examples of habitual barriers and insights from students.

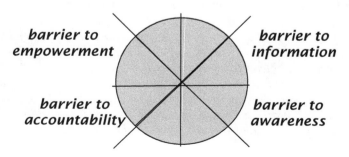

Barriers to Information are habits people have which interfere with their ability to gather, understand, and use information about ethics and about power. These habits include getting continually confused, choosing not to read a code at all, or dismissing or disregarding information.

These habits are held in place by beliefs such as:

- *"I'm a good person, therefore I won't cause any harm."*
- *"I don't need rules. I'll use my common sense and my integrity.*
- *"If I find out about the guidelines, I'm afraid I might discover I've done something wrong."*
- *"I just don't understand what all this emphasis on ethics is all-about."*
- *"I don't want to buy into the whole system."*
- *"I already know all these things."*
- *"I only trust my own inner guidance."*
- *"I'm just too busy doing the WORK!"*
- *"Codes for someone else--for idealists."*

After personal exploration of this aspect, participants have said

- *"I don't want to abuse my power by under-using it ever again."*
- *"I want to now actively nourish the right use of my power."*
- *"I now understand how and why I stop myself from knowing and the reason is fear."*
- *"Thinking of ethics codes as lived wisdom is inspiring. I see them in a different way now."*

Barriers to awareness seem to organize around shame or fear of being overwhelmed by the pain of remembering old wounds of power. Habits that interfere with increasing awareness include numbing, disconnecting from the heart, and discounting experience.

Beliefs such as:

- *"If I remember, I'll never stop crying."*
- *"I was so hurt, I decided I'd never risk being powerful because I might hurt someone else."*
- *"I'll be overwhelmed by shame."*
- *"It's too risky to know too much."*
- *"I need to protect people from my power."*
- *"No one will get to me again."*
- *"When my power is generated through love, I'm safe."*

Unburdening through stories and these barriers and beliefs, participants have gained insights such as

- *"Power is a feedback loop for self-knowledge."*
- *"I can be humble in my power."*
- *"I have a feeling in my bones that I don't have to be ashamed, ambivalent, or hide my power anymore."*
- *"I'm ready to claim my history differently."*

Barriers to accountability are imbued with fear, shame, or paranoia and are associated with beliefs such as:

- *"It's not my fault."*
- *"If I apologize for anything, it will be used against me."*
- *"They're making all this up."*
- *"I did the best I could."*
- *"I never said that at all."*
- *"My client is resistant and defensive."*
- *"It wasn't my intention to cause harm."*
- *"I'm a good person and I'm being victimized."*
- *"It doesn't matter what I do, it doesn't work."*
- *"It's always gonna be my fault."*
- *"I've got it handled. If I take action, I'll get hurt."*

These are reflected in habits of being defensive, accusing or blaming the other, not responding at all, hoping it will all go away on it's own, poor assessment of your actual power (either more or less), or keeping secrets.

Working with the material in this aspect, participants have said such things as

- *"I see that I can get better at using difficulties to clarify, resolve, or deepen my connections, instead of avoiding conflict. It's a complete reframe on conflict."*
- *"I can be forgiven and be resourced by my goodness instead of my shame."*
- *"I need to allow myself to make mistakes before I can allow others to."*

Barriers to empowerment seem to center around fear of one's potential for goodness (or harm).

- *"If I do well this time, people will expect me to be perfect."*

- *"I don't want to be seen as arrogant."*
- *"We're all equal here. I don't have power over anyone."*
- *"What I'm doing is just a little thing, not skillful use of power."*
- *"If I use my power, I'll be visible and get attacked."*
- *"I'm afraid to step up and be a leader."*

These attitudes are reflected in habits of disowning power, not fully showing up, over-focusing on personal wounds and suffering, not taking a stand, giving up, not letting go, not developing skill and vision.

Practitioners have discovered such things as
- *"I will use my power to create my life."*
- *"I am now confident that I can use my power with love."*
- *"I don't have to wait until I'm not scared to begin. I can use my fear to remind myself of my integrity and sensitivity."*
- *"I am learning to recognize when to let go of something."*

Right Use of Power teacher, Conway Weary summarizes the challenges as differences between right use and misuse of power in a chart--consciously over-simplified but useful.

right uses of power		misuses of power
in information, compassion, connection	*originate*	in ignorance, fear, subjugation, domination, greed, disconnection
consciously	*are applied*	unconsciously or sometimes consciously
sensitivity, self-awareness, accountability, feedback, collaboration, resolution and repair	*use*	poor or no sensitivity, self-awareness, accountability, feedback, collaboration, resolution or repair
increased skill, satisfaction, enhanced relationships	*result in*	wounding, exploitation, disempowerment, desire for revenge

Shadow Effects of Elevated Power

In the light of day, we all have shadows: aspects of ourselves that are hidden from our sight unless we look directly at them. Often our friends and colleagues can see our shadow even when we can't. Here's another challenge to using power sensitively and wisely: power has its own nature, with good and bad effects.

Research by Joris Lammers, Dacher Keltner and others, is showing that people who have increased power act differently from people who have lesser power. This is true whether the elevated power comes from role or status. Increased or decreased power has cognitive, behavioral, emotional, and somatic effects. "Good" people tend to have the idea that those who abuse their up-power do so because they are simply greedy, fearful, self-aggrandizing, or power-hungry. However, it turns out that the situation is more complicated. Power affects everyone, and unless it is understood and mediated, it results in abuses. In fact, the greater the power difference, the greater and more widespread the harm. The widely held idea (Lord Acton) that "power corrupts and absolute power corrupts absolutely" is largely true.

There are gifts and there are perils of power and they affect everyone in high power roles no matter what their intention. Like the ring of power in *Lord of the Rings*, when you put on the ring of role and/or status power you, you are affected and challenged. Even Frodo, the pure, had tremendous trouble resisting the pull of the ring to being self-serving, greedy, possessed. Increased role power is a change agent. It changes how you see yourself, how you see others, and how they see you. So, what are these effects, and what kind of self-reinforcing loop do these effects create?

1. **Social distance.** The gift of social distance is that it allows a leader to see from a larger perspective and thus make informed decisions for the greatest good for the greatest number, even though not all those affected may be happy with the decision. The shadow impacts of social distance, however, are many and perilous. Those with greater power can and are likely to dehumanize those down-power to them by seeing them as objects that are expendable and can be dominated and exploited. Soldiers are unable to kill unless they dehumanize their enemy. A Nazi officer reported receiving "1000 Jew pieces at the station" and disposing of them. Sadly, those with increased social distance linked with their elevated power become less empathic, more dehumanizing, more self-sufficient, less aware of the impact of their actions, and less likely to offer support and help.

2. **Freedom to act with no or limited interference**. The gift of this effect is that it enables the person in the up-power role to take charge, making decisions quickly when action is necessary. The shadow of this effect causes those with greater power to be impulsive and unconstrained; inappropriate with touch, flirting and teasing; interruptive and more aggressive and disrespectful; less vigilant, and to fail to understand other's

needs and desires. They ignore, are unaffected by or punish those who offer critical feedback. Increased power also causes leaders to have stricter standards for others than for themselves and to stick to the rules regardless of whether they have negative or positive impacts. They use shame, pathologizing, harrassing and humiliation to stay in control. They also shift the blame for their mistakes and misuses of power onto others with lower power.

   3. **You become larger than you are**. With the addition of role power you become larger than your personal self. As a leader you can use this gift for important and effective influence. However, the perils are many. Leaders tend to identify with their increased power as if it were their personal power rather than added-on role power that comes with responsibilities and opportunities for care and effectiveness. Such a misunderstanding of who they truly are results in deep disconnection from empathic, respectful, and sustainable relationships. On the opposite end of the continuum, when leaders try to disown or downplay their up-power role, they cause harm by being unable to use their role power to provide protection and promote the common good. In addition, they become the object for projections of images and expectations associated with the role that may lead to either being idealized or devalued. The temptation is strong to get personal needs for love, money, sex, control inappropriately met through the power of role or rank.

   4. **You have access to greater resources and opportunities**. Obviously, this gift supports those in up-power roles in carrying out their responsibilities effectively and with the resources they need. However, leaders tend to fall under the spell of perks and privileges, like gifts, tickets to events, special favors. They also tend to lose awareness of their limitations and prioritize their own needs. Because of the emotional and behavioral changes associated with elevated power, higher power individuals take actions that prioritize their own needs and act freely on their whims. While those with lower power have an avoidance orientation. They take actions to avoid punishment or loss and to placate the leader.

   Not surprisingly, the attitudes and behaviors resulting from the effects of greater power create a self-reinforcing harmful loop of exploitation and abuse. The horrific way that power's shadow plays itself out in the world would have those who want to be helpful and leave the world a better place running away from power. However, as much as anything else, we need people who will say "yes" to their elevated role power and learn to use it sensitively and humbly. Accepting leadership and role power with wisdom and compassion is not for the faint of heart. Doing so takes courage and skill.   It seems important to stop for a moment and feel compassion for all human beings when we are in up-power roles. May we respond to the call to understand and mediate the shadow effects.

Here's the good news.   By understanding these normal effects of power, we can bring them out of the shadows and into the light. When we shine a light on them, we can choose to take action to mediate or decrease these negative effects. And here's more good news.   These effects are cognitive, emotional, and behavioral tendencies.   Research shows that people with a moral center made up of attitudes and values such as kindness, humility, honesty, respect and fairness, are much less affected by the shadow effects of elevated power.[ccix] Information about these shadow effects is valuable when in an up-power role because it enables you to be vigilant and pro-active. This information is also valuable when in a down-power role because, knowing the methods being used by those who are u-power, you can, as a result, be more empowered and strategic in your responses.

We have the stunning opportunity to change Lord Acton's insight from power <u>always</u> corrupts to power <u>can</u> corrupt. Understanding, vigilance, and skill can prevent power differences from becoming abusive and keep relationships healthy. We can restore compassion to the dynamic between up- and down-power roles: authority with collaboration, strength with heart.

The deepest impact of the shadow effects of power is disconnection: the inability or unwillingness to experience the negative effects of one's actions. Right relationship is built on a foundation of empathy. Empathy is not possible when there is no connection. The greater the power difference, the further the relationship distance, and the harder it is to feel for those in your care. The best antidote for the negative impacts of power is staying in or returning to right relationship. In my experience right relationship has two aspects. Both have to do with empathy. One is staying in empathic connection with the people who are in down-power roles. The other is having and maintaining a vision or mission that is larger than egotistic self-interest, fear, and the need for control.   This vision is driven by compassion for the well-being of all and for being and staying in right relationship with others.

Four recommendations for managing your power shadow

1. BE INFORMED. Own your role power and its inherent responsibilities and opportunities and be vigilant for the shadow of your power.

2. BE AWARE. Strive to be humble, know your strengths and limitations and stay in touch with your center pole and moral compass.

3. BE CONNECTED. Stay present and connected with both strength and heart to those in your care and, at the same time, to yourself. Remember the 150% principle and have confidence in your ability to resolve and repair.

4. BE SKILLFUL. Elicit and use feedback well. Be pro-active about your ethical edges. Know how to self-reflect, self-correct, apologize, and forgive.

Stand in your power and stay in your heart.

Self-study: Exploring Challenges

1. Barriers
Move reflectively around the Power Spiral and think about, journal, or talk with a partner about four things:
1. Mistakes you might be vulnerable to making because of your habits at each barrier.
2. Things you have learned or understood from this book related to each aspect of the power spiral.
3. An example of your right use of power in this aspect. (Don't be surprised if you discover that acknowledging your competence is more difficult than acknowledging your woundedness or mistakes.)

4. Inner or outer resources you have or are available to you to support your ethical sensitivity and accountability at these barriers.

2. Old Story/New Story

1. As you read the common beliefs for each barrier, notice which one's "ding" as beliefs of yours. Is there a different one that encapsulates your barrier? *("I have no power.")*

2. Choose one of these negative beliefs. Find a sentence or a gesture that triggers this belief (your Old Story). *(Turning away and looking distracted.)*

3. If you have a partner, instruct your partner to do the gesture or say the sentence you have just named, even though you don't believe it. *(Turning away and looking distracted.)* Notice what happens in your body when you are experiencing your Old Story. *(It feels like my body shrinks. I feel young and small and I shut down inside.)*

4. Now then, what would you like the New Story to be? State this new story as a belief. *(I have power and I can own it.)*

5. If you are working with a partner, have your partner say the New Story to you. *(You have power and you can own it.)* Notice what happens in your body when you try on this New Story. *(I feel bigger and more upright. It feels good.)*

6. Now have your partner say the sentence or do the gesture that triggers the Old Story *(Turning away and looking distracted)* while you embody the new story. What do you notice? *(It's almost funny. I feel unaffected. Like the looking away isn't about me at all. I can stay here and connect.)*

7. Have your partner say the New Story while you are embodying the New Story.

8. Rock back and forth between the two postures to deepen your felt sense of the shift you may want to make. You may be surprised about the shift that happens. You can experience a major shift in belief and response instantly, however, integrating this New Belief into your life will most likely take some time. Think about how this shift will positively affect your ethical awareness and decision-making.

3. Limitations

Fold a big sheet of newsprint in half and make a drawing of your leadership limitations on one side of the fold and your leadership resources on the other side. When your drawing is complete, open the paper up and notice and explore the relationship between the two sides.

4. Growing Edge

Being pro-active on your own behalf and actively using a support and professional consultation network are two of the most important actions you can take to be ethically responsible.

Make and write down an assessment of your possible vulnerabilities:

A. In relationship to the specific guidelines of your profession's code of ethics.

B. From assessing how well your needs are being met in the following three areas:

Financial / Social / Intimacy

And how strong your needs are for:

Love & Approval / Being Right / Control / Intensity

Areas of unmet needs or over-focused motivation are places where you may be particularly vulnerable to unconsciousness and mistakes. *(Of course, these desires are normal and not to be denied, but understood and self-corrected when they are out of balance.)*

Some examples:

    • *Unmet financial needs could lead to unconsciously continuing to work with clients longer than is needed.*

    • *Unmet social needs could lead to getting involved in inappropriate or unmanaged dual roles.*

    • *Unmet intimacy needs could lead to inappropriate use of touch or sexual involvement or innuendo.*

    • *Very strong needs for love and approval could lead to not being willing to keep agreements about paying for missed sessions.*

    • *Very strong needs to be right could lead to difficulty in acknowledging your client's experience when it is different from yours.*

    • *Very strong needs for control could lead to the use of unnecessary force.*

    • *Very strong needs for intensity could lead to an over-focus on the drama of disturbing events or areas of dysfunction.*

5. Secrets

Are there any secrets you've been keeping about unethical behavior? Under what circumstances would it be necessary, useful, or important to share this? Are you responsible for any harm that needs repair? Is there a way to repair it?" Note that you may have secrets about misuses of both up-power and down-power.

6. Sustainers and Drainers

Make a list of things that help sustain you in using your power wisely and well and on the other side of the sheet list things that drain you. *(For example, sustainer: being in the presence of others using their power well, drainer: being over-tired, or being in a dominating or humiliating environment.)*

"An enemy is one whose story we haven't yet heard."
—*Gene Hoffman*[ccx]

"Nearly all men can stand adversity, but if you want to test a man's character, give him power."
—*Abraham Lincoln*

The Parable of the Thorns   —*May Shaw Gale*[ccxi]
Bless the road that is afflicted with thorns,
for it requires a mindful step
and an eye for the open spaces in between
where one might skillfully
slip toward the freedom
of the golden meadow ahead.
Where lapses of focus
bring sharp wounds
that, of themselves,
might teach the feet a surer step
or even inspire a small retreat,
a place to catch one's breath and reconnect
to Earth and Heart and Faith.
Where the prickly lessons of compassion
are dispensed, sometimes
with drops of blood,
but send the traveler on her path
with an expanded view of the sky above.

Soul Work & World Service

"We need an ethic of compassion more desperately than ever before."   —*Karen Armstrong, reflecting on the unanimous agreement of religious faiths on the primacy of compassion*[ccxii]

"We are not here to save the world, we are here to love and serve the world and in that love and in that service, the world may or may not be saved."   —*Gurumai*[ccxiii]

"The final piece of reaching for authentic power is releasing your own to a higher form of wisdom."   —*Gary Zukov*[ccxiv]

"Pain and suffering, they are a mystery. Kindness and love, they are a mystery. But I have learned that kindness and love can pay for pain and suffering."   —*Barbara Kingsolver*[ccxv]

Weaving ethics with soul work and with world service is a natural outgrowth of understanding ethics as right use of the power of love and the power of influence.

There are several colored threads to this weaving:

* The development of skillfulness and wisdom in the benevolent use of power combined with the force of love requires personal and relationship work at the level of soul.
* One of the characteristics of health and well-being is altruistic desire and action.
* Clients may need guidance and support, as their well-being improves, in putting their compassion and benevolence into action in the world.
* The growth and expression of compassion is as primary as self-esteem in happiness and health.[ccxvi]

"The force of love is the same as the force of the soul or truth. We have evidence of its working at every step. The universe would disappear without the existence of that force. But you ask for historical evidence. It is, therefore, necessary to know what "history" means. If it means the doings of kings and emperors, how they became enemies of one another, how they murdered one another, and if this were all that had happened in the world, it would have been ended long ago. Little quarrels in millions of families in their daily lives disappear before the exercise of this force. Hundreds of nations live in peace. History does not and cannot take note of this fact. History is really a record of every interruption of the even working of the force of love or of the soul. Soul force, being natural, is not noted in history."[ccxvii]   —Gandhi*

Altruism and the Soul

"Altruism is a natural expression of human development and a healing force in society...Caring coupled with imagination and enterprise is the essence of creative altruism. If we ignore our capacity for compassion and care, we diminish the texture of our lives, our ability to help others heal and grow, and our collective potentials for social healing. By opening ourselves to the reality of shared being, we enhance the wonder and richness of the world and liberate the creative and constructive energies of the human heart, mind, and spirit."[ccxviii]   —Tom Hurley*

Karen Armstrong adds to her statement about the need for an ethic of compassion: *"The early prophets did not preach the discipline of empathy because it sounded edifying, but because experience showed that it worked. They discovered that greed and selfishness were the cause of our personal misery. When we gave them up, we were happier. Egotism imprisoned us in an inferior version of ourselves and impeded our enlightenment."*[ccxix] Fascinatingly, recent neurological research by Moll and Jordan Grafman has shown that taking action in the best interests of others is coded in the brain. In a study in which they scanned the "brains of volunteers as they were asked to think about a scenario involving either donating a sum of money to charity or keeping it for themselves," the results showed that "when the volunteers placed the interests of others before their own, the generosity activated a primitive part of the brain that usually lights up in response to food or sex. Altruism, the experiment suggested, was not a superior moral faculty that suppresses basic selfish urges, but rather was basic to the brain, hard-wired and pleasurable."[ccxx] There is a surviving and thriving impulse and advantage for those who develop and use their capacities for social intelligence. This social intelligence is accessed through the social engagement nervous system referred to on page 117).

Compassion, not selectively for those who are similar—for that is easy—but for those who are different, even 'enemies,' is what brings, not only greater happiness and spiritual development, but also peaceful relations and the sustaining prosperity that comes from mutual aid. Compassion for all simply works better than aggression. Right use of power comes from compassion for all, rather than from fearful aggression.

Because it feels good, because it makes us happier, because it improves relationships, because it makes the world a better place—for all these reasons, we need to support the soul development of compassion for all, including ourselves.

Story: My psychotherapy client sat down, took a moment and said, "I don't think there's anything to work on today." "Maybe so. Why don't you take a little time quietly with yourself and see if your unconscious offers something up to us out of the inner space you create, and if not, you could just leave for today." After about five minutes, Margie said, "There is something kind of peeking out. It's an impulse to do something to help on a world level." "That sounds like health. You've been healing and empowering yourself. The desire for altruism is an organic thing. What's it like when you experience this impulse peeking out?" "It's like I feel like a child...very small, looking up at all these big, powerful people in high government positions." "Overwhelmed and insignificant?" "Yes, and very naïve. Like, I've been in such a small little world, isolated. I guess I've been trying to keep my life manageable and safe." "So you're scared when you open up to a larger world." "Yes, and then I have all these questions....How do I find reliable sources of information...I'm so uninformed. How do I not get overwhelmed by all the pain and disasters? How do I find some way to help that would be effective and not too painful or draining?" "Lots of good questions." "Too big, I can't sustain this impulse...it just goes away."

How do we help our clients and ourselves channel the natural impulse for altruism? How do we help them discover that service is a primary source of contentment and meaning? What is the curriculum for the soul work of learning compassion? Karen Armstrong's curriculum is simple. She tells a *Story: "Rabbi Hillel, the older contemporary of Jesus, taught the golden rule in a particularly emphatic way. One day a heathen asked him to sum up the whole of Jewish teaching while standing on one leg.*

Hillel stood on one leg and replied: "that which is hateful to you, do not do to your neighbor. That is the Torah; the rest is commentary; go and learn it!"[ccxxi] The practice of right use of power and influence goes beyond the treatment room. This is ethics as world service.

Humility

When you say yes to the responsibilities and opportunities of an up-power role, when you humbly remember that this additional power is role-embedded, and when you seek to use your power with wisdom and skill, you automatically access a kind of guidance, energy, and information that is available through the role.

In my first years of being a therapist and then of teaching, I was quite nervous and fearful that I wouldn't know enough or be good enough. Over time, I became aware and learned to trust that I would, by owning and saying yes to my role, receive information and guidance from somewhere beyond me.

Moral (Ethical) Development

Ethical use of power begins in empathy and altruistic pleasure. We are born with a basic moral compass, based in empathy and the natural desire to take action on behalf of others. This is most obvious in the outpouring of care for a family member or a situation in which one is directly involved. Simple moral decisions activate a straightforward brain response. The Snyders have spent a lifetime studying young children as persons. They have consistently found that children have an inborn pre-disposition for justice and caring. "Unless they have been dehumanized by adults . . . children reveal the capacity to be empathically attuned to each other, to co-create a 'justice culture,' to support fairness, safety and the restoration of relationship, and to be naturally interested in what works for the well-being of all."[ccxxii] This is what we would expect from our brain wiring. Of course, when this brain wiring in the frontal lobes is damaged or inoperative, people suffer from a complete lack of empathy and conscience, clinically labeled psychopathy.[ccxxiii] While not all who meet the definition of psychopath are violent, they live with a lack of the normal empathy and conscience that guides behavior. When in leadership positions, and they are there, these people are particularly difficult if not impossible to deal with.

Our brains are hard-wired for empathic responses toward the well-being of others. There is global agreement about basic human rights, in theory at least elucidated in detail in the U.N. Universal Declaration of

Human Rights, reprinted in the Appendix. There are virtues common to descriptions of what qualities are important to being a good person in the core teachings of major world religions. Linda Kavelin and Dan Popov identified 52 of these through studying the texts of the world's great religions.[ccxxiv]Karen Armstrong recently proposed the creation of a contract for compassion to be signed by the leaders of world religions.[ccxxv] Global agreement on top values of honesty, responsibility, respect, and fairness exists.[ccxxvi] Clear situations where there is a choice to alleviate suffering, like picking up a hurt child, giving money to support victims of a fire, sharing food with someone who is hungry, activate a straightforward brain response.

Other situations are more complex and activate competing brain center activity, like abortion, euthanasia, population control, and use of global resources. Here's where the life long process of moral and ethical development begins.

There are many moral development theories. I'll mention several here. Lawrence Kohlberg, who delineated the classic theory of stages and levels, identifies developmental perceptions of rules and of what "right" is. Oversimplifying his system, rules are to be obeyed to avoid punishment; then rules are to be followed in order not to cause harm; and then rules are seen as beneficial and can be changed if they are unfair. "Right" is first seen as satisfying one's own needs; then as doing one's duty and respecting authority; and then right is an integrated and organic expression of concern for all in a given situation.[ccxxvii] Knowledge of these developmental and perceptual differences has potential value in fine-tuning your skills in dealing with clients, colleagues and superiors who may be guided by different perceptions, especially in talking about ethical codes and the concept of right use of power.

Carol Gilligan, another theorist, using Kohlberg's model, found that in their moral development, men tend to operate from an ethic of justice while women operate from an ethic of care. While Kohlberg puts focus on justice as a higher stage than a focus on care, Gilligan considers these a same level difference between boys and girls. Gilligan says, "An ethic of justice proceeds from the premise of equality—that all should be treated the same," while "an ethic of care rests on the premise of non-violence—that no one should be harmed."[ccxxviii] The flavor of this difference seems to be reflected in the difference in perspective between relationship prudence (as seen in mediation and restorative justice programs) and jurisprudence (as seen in most grievance processes and in legal actions.) The right use of power model advocated here is a meld of the two concerns—for justice, and for care—power with heart.

Ken Wilber speaks of evolution as proceeding by including and yet transcending what went before. Both he and Gilligan would agree that moral and ethical development proceeds in this fashion. Moral development is seen as a hierarchical in that "each stage has a higher capacity for care and compassion."[ccxxix]Stage 1 is labeled **egocentric**— morality is centered on "me". Including and transcending, by Stage 2 called **ethnocentric**, a person's identity now extends to members of their group, i.e. community, family, religious affiliation, school. At Stage 3 **world centric** another inclusion and expansion has taken place and care and compassion is felt and expressed toward all of humanity. Gilligan follows development further in describing the highest stage of moral development, which she calls **integrated**, as a 4th stage in which the voices of the masculine and feminine, the voices for justice and the voices for compassion, become integrated.[ccxxx]It is clear that at the egocentric stage, moral decisions are relatively simple and black and white. Parents and teachers know that children feel empathy and can act on behalf of others. However, as we expand into the ethnocentric, world centric and integrated stages, ethical sensitivity, awareness, and decision-making becomes more and more complex and challenging. These higher levels of development what I consider the soul work of using power with heart.

I see ethical development as occurring in a spiraling fashion, as in the power spiral described in this book—moral development spiraling through the four dimensions. Ken Wilber speaks of development unfolding in 4 quadrants (4 fundamental perspectives), which seem akin to the 4 dimensions in the right use of power model. Wilber's 4 quadrants[ccxxxi] roughly correspond to the 4 dimensions perspectives (see pages 10-11 for more detail) as follows:

4 Quadrants	**4 Dimensions**
"I" (the inside of the individual)	Self (Be Compassionate)
"It" (the outside of the individual)	Guidance (Be Informed)
"We" (the inside of the collective)	Relationship (Be Connected)
"Its" (the outside of the collective)	Wisdom (Be Skillful)

I hope the power spiral model will provide both guidance and a framework for ethical soul work leading to effective and wise world service.

The Power Paradox

Given that brain research and universal religious values support basic goodness and natural altruism, why is it that there is so much misuse and abuse of power? This is a question I have been tracking since I was a youngster at camp and I became very distressed and just could not understand why one of my tent-mates had stolen another camper's comic books.

This is a question that has also concerned Dr. Dacher Keltner, a professor of psychology at the University of California. He has done considerable research about who gets power and how they use it once they get it. It seems we have been *"guided by centuries of advice from Machiavelli" and more recently "from Robert Greene's The 48 Laws of Power, (for example: Conceal Your Intentions, Use Selective Honesty and Generosity to Disarm Your Victims, Crush Your Enemy Totally, Keep Others in Suspended Terror, Always Say Less than Necessary, Court Attention at all Cost, and Do Not Commit to Anyone) to tend to believe that attaining power requires force, deception, manipulation, and coercion. Indeed, we might even assume that positions of power demand this kind of conduct-that to run smoothly, society needs leaders who are willing and able to use power this way."*[ccxxxii]

New research on power, supported by brain research on hard-wired morality referred to earlier in this chapter, reveals, however, that *"power is wielded most effectively when it's used responsibly, by people who are attuned to and engaged with the needs and interests of others. Years of research suggests that empathy and social intelligence are vastly more important to acquiring and exercising power than are force, deception, or terror. [However,] studies also show that once people assume positions of power, they're likely to act more selfishly, impulsively, and aggressively, and they have a harder time seeing the world from other people's points of view. This presents us with the paradox of power: The skills most important to obtaining power and leading effectively are the very skills that deteriorate once we have power."*[ccxxxiii]

Naming and understanding this power paradox is of great importance to the soul work of right use of power advocated here. When in positions of power, we are in positions in which we are on the up-power side of the power differential. Knowing that research shows that in these positions, we are more vulnerable to misusing power, we need to increase our sensitivity, and vigilance about continuing to use our power rightly.

The research is interesting. *"Highly detailed studies of 'chimpanzee politics' have found that social power among non-human primates is based less on sheer strength, coercion, and the unbridled assertion of self-interest, and more on the ability to negotiate conflicts, to enforce group norms, and to allocate resources fairly."*[ccxxxiv] Dacher Keltner's research shows similar results with human social hierarchies. In research about social hierarchies within college dormitories, the researchers *"made the*

*remarkable discovery that modesty may be critical to maintaining power.
Individuals who are modest about their own power actually rise in
hierarchies and maintain the status and respect of their peers, while
individuals with an inflated, grandiose sense of power quickly fall to the
bottom rungs....[In addition,] people instinctively identify individuals who
might undermine the interest of the group, and prevent those people from
rising in power, through what we call 'reputational discourse.'"* ccxxxv So
cultivation and use of social intelligence, i.e. modesty, empathy,
engagement with the needs of others, and skill in negotiating conflicts,
enforcing norms, and allocating resources fairly is not only right use of
power but important to both gaining and maintaining power.

Now let's look at the research about the other side of the power
paradox. Research shows that *"power leads people to act in impulsive
fashion, both good and bad, and to fail to understand other people's
feelings and desires . . . For instance, studies have found that people given
power in experiments are more likely to rely on stereotypes when judging
others, and they pay less attention to the characteristics that define those
other people as individuals. Predisposed to stereotype, they also judge
others' attitudes, interests, and needs less accurately. . . Power
encourages individuals to act on their own whims, desires, and impulses.
When researchers give people power in scientific experiments, those
people are more likely to physically touch others in potentially
inappropriate ways, to flirt in more direct fashion, [and] to make risky
choices and gambles . . . Perhaps more unsettling is the wealth of evidence
that having power makes people more likely to. . . .interrupt others, to
speak out of turn, and to fail to look at others who are speaking . . .Surveys
of organizations find that most rude behaviors—shouting, profanities, bald
critiques—emanate from the offices. . . .of individuals in positions of
power."* ccxxxvi

Once again, here's the power paradox: *"Power is given to those
individuals, groups, or nations who advance the interests of the greater
good in socially-intelligent fashion. Yet, unfortunately, having power
renders many individuals. . . .impulsive and poorly attuned to others . . .
making them prone to act abusively and lose the esteem of their peers.
What people want from leaders—social intelligence—is what is damaged
by the experience of power."* ccxxxvii

What factors would begin to explain this odd paradox? Here's my
sense of it.   **1)** Because of the impact of the power differential, those in
up-power role are **removed and remove themselves from the checks and
balances of the feedback loop** in which people tell each other either
directly or indirectly about their impact both positive and negative. When

in down-power position, it is perceived and may truly be too risky to offer negative feedback. The up-power persons then don't hear the negatives and either or both lose their ability to reality check and feel immune to the usual consequences of abuse of power. **2)** People tend to over-identify with their power role, **experiencing their enhanced power as entirely personal rather than role power.** This leads to grandiosity and an unrealistic sense of Self. **3)** People in up-power are also **embedded in systems in which it is difficult to act alone** and which become invisible to those in the system. These systems support or even mandate particular behaviors that may contribute to right or wrong uses of power. Systems are very complex because members usually are aware of only one or several pieces of the system. **4)** We have **socially conditioned expectations and misconceptions about the use of power.** We have long been accustomed to thinking of power as manipulation, undue force, coercion, terror, and deception. We have understood that that was what power was, how it was earned, and how it was effective. And so, we have put up with this model of power and sanctioned it, even though it causes egregious harm. Now is the time to change our model of power.

Changing our personal and collective expectations about right use of power to one that embodies social intelligence and links power with heart is truly ethics as soul work. Movement toward this change will happen through: 1) Owning your personal and professional power as the vital ability to use power to prevent harm, reduce harm, repair harm, and promote well-being; 2) Campaigning for a socially-responsible model of power; 3) Developing and using your skills for actively participating in the feedback loop; 4) Becoming more and more sensitive to your impact especially when in power differential positions; 5) Strategically and skillfully stopping expecting, condoning, or feeling helpless about misuses of power in systems and up-power individuals. Begin to expect and require social intelligence. This is right use of soul power.

The Soul of Service

Rachel Naomi Remen[ccxxxviii] hones the experience and value to both others and to ourselves in these excerpts in which she distinguishes service from helping or fixing. *"We serve with ourselves. We draw from all of our experiences. Our limitations serve, our wounds serve, and even our darkness can serve. The wholeness in us serves the wholeness in others and the wholeness in me...Service...is an experience of mystery, surrender, and awe...A server knows that he or she is being used and has a willingness to be used in the service of something greater, something essentially unknown...Everyone who has ever served through the history of time serves the same thing. We are servers of the wholeness and mystery of life. The bottom line, of course, is that we can fix without serving. And we can help without serving. And we can serve without fixing or helping. I think I would go so far as to say that fixing and helping may often be the work of the ego, and service the work of the soul...Our service serves us as well as others. That which uses us strengthens us. Over time, fixing and helping are draining, depleting. Over time we burn out. Service is renewing. When we can serve, our work itself will sustain us."*

> *"I slept and dreamt that life was joy;*
> *I awoke and saw that life was service;*
> *I acted and behold, service was joy."*
> *—Rabindranath Tagore*[ccxxxix]

Joanna Macy[ccxl] speaks of a pair of wings. *"I resonate with Carl Jung when he says that a central shift in our time is from seeing spirituality as a journey toward perfection, to seeing it as a journey toward wholeness. To my mind, that changes everything. It even feels like a different posture. Instead of holding aloof from travail to clutch and climb up a ladder to the sacred, the movement is to open the arms and embrace it right here."* Coming from a Buddhist perspective, she says, *"The two wings on which the bodhisattva flies are compassion and wisdom. Instead of looking for a safe harbor, for a place where you're all protected and cozy and safe, you just fly high on these two wings and place your trust in them. We need both of them: compassion, and insight into the radical interdependence of all phenomena. One isn't enough. We need the compassion because that openness to the pain of the world provides the fuel to move you out where you need to be, to do what you need to do. Yes, compassion by itself, without understanding and trusting our interconnectedness, can burn you out. So you need the other wing, the wisdom that knows how interwoven we are in the web of life, inseparable from each other. That wisdom reminds us that we're not involved in a battle between good guys and bad guys, for the line between good and evil runs through the landscape of every human heart. ...But wisdom by itself is not enough to move us forward for the sake of all beings; it needs the steady, heart-opening beat of compassion. Then we fly."*

Making Soul Connections

Many people feel that a soul connection between therapist and client must be made before healing, safety, and trust can happen. Assagioli is said to have stated: *"Therapy is what happens while two souls connect."* This could be true for other forms of healing work. Bodyworkers might add their belief that the body is the clearest vessel of the soul. Another way to put this is to say that the healing relationship can be a crucible in which souls connect and that the power of healing is in this very connection. Others experience healing as an organic process waiting for a place to happen. What is your point of view?

Resources for the Soul

Having access to sources of spiritual nourishment, support, courage and perspective is a deep resource for the soul work of Right Use of Power. For those engaged in using power in world service, spiritual resourcing is essential to the sustaining of the work. There are, of course, many, many sources of spiritual support.

Gandhi's[ccxli] words inspire:

> *"Victory is in the doing, not the results."*
> *"We must be the change we want to see in the world."*
> *"It is best to work for love and not against evil."*

Angeles Arrien[ccxlii] offers a resourcing question and process that I have adapted: Ask yourself, What is the resource I need to support my wise and skillful use of power? Go to a place of mindfulness and ask it to reveal itself to you. Then image placing this resource before you, behind you, to the left of you, to the right of you, and around you.

I have also found it to be spiritually resourcing when I feel despairing or obsessed with doing—to feel myself as a drop of water and then let myself expand to feel my connection to an ocean of like-minded souls.

Four-Fold Way

Angeles Arrien's *Four-Fold Way* informs and resources the power spiral. Refer to the graphic at the beginning of Dimension Four.

Right Use of Power as soul work in the Four-Fold Way
   Guided: Show Up
   Conscious: Pay attention to what has heart and meaning
   Responsible: Tell and hear the truth without shame or blame
   Wise: Be open to outcome, not attached to outcome

Two purposes: vertical and horizontal

My friend Elizabeth Cogburn[ccxliii] talks about having two purposes in her lifetime: a Vertical Purpose that she describes as spiritual purpose, soul work, "being" aspect of Self; and a Horizontal Purpose meaning community world service, political activities, world work, the "doing" aspect of Self. This vertical/horizontal purpose distinction is what is referred to in the title of this topic: Soul Work and World Service.

One of the great tasks is to find ways to bring these two together, like a circle scribed with a horizontal and a vertical line or making sure you are flying with both wings unfurled—the wing of vertical purpose, and the wing of horizontal purpose. Together, these two purposes "grow corn"—tangible, nourishing, sustaining fruit.

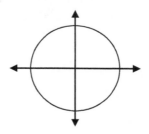

Ethics and Soul Work

"In the world at present, there is not much concern for humane values; there is too much dependence on money and power. If human society loses the value of honesty, we will face greater difficulties in the future. Some people may think that these sorts of ethical attitudes are not much needed in the areas of business or politics. I strongly disagree. The quality of our actions depends on our motivation. What we must do is to balance external material progress with the sense of responsibility that comes of education and inner development." —*The Dalai Lama*[ccxliv]

Right Use of Power is the biggest container for ethics since it includes social consciousness and personal development. In this greatest context, ethics is about reverence for life, treating all people with respect, and acting honorably.

This context includes and honors the value of prescribed codes and guidelines and goes beyond into the realm of repairing harm, restoring relationships, and promoting well-being. Ethical behavior in this framework requires a high level of consciousness development and understanding of both harm and empowerment.

Ken Wilber speaks of evolutionary consciousness development as a de-centering process where each level transcends, yet includes the previous stage, like concentric rings of a circle, each expanding the number of perspectives that one can empathically and compassionately hold, accept, and honor without prejudice. From allegiance to self as center, we expand our consciousness to family, to community or religion, to country, to world, to a transcendental perspective.

Ethics at the level of soul work asks from us:

1. On-going personal and spiritual work.
2. An ability to be authentic and, at the same time, be in service to other(s).
3. The humility to know and take responsibility when we've made a mistake or inadvertently caused harm.
4. A level of transcendence in which we can put our own needs aside in order to be of service.
5. Access to a sense of unity and oneness.
6. An ability to foster independence even when we're being depended upon for our helpfulness.
7. Thorough knowledge of Self and an ability to use our strengths as resources and minimize the impact of our vulnerabilities.
8. A capacity to be in the presence of suffering and woundedness with compassion and without dissociating, numbing, or getting overwhelmed.
9. A calling to "make real" our gifts and intentions.
10. A willingness to have influence.

Conscious Evolution

Barbara Marx Hubbard[ccxlv] has a vision of an evolutionary leap from individual spiritual development to attunement within the field of consciousness. We have the capacity to raise our sensitivity to be able to resonate with this field. Once attuned to this all-encompassing field of awareness and love, we can co-create what manifests in the world, keeping in mind that patterns of good most likely have other ways of manifesting than through human beings. Her position is that nature is good, but it is not kind, and that we are the ones who can bring kindness into evolution. Human-<u>kind</u>. She reminds that by 1945 we had gained powers we used to attribute to God, like, instant destruction, instant communication across space, predicting weather, and curing diseases. We now must use these powers with love, or we will self-destruct. We need a consciousness of the heart in addition to a consciousness of the mind.

To be a leader of the heart, her prescription is to let go of your small success agenda in service of a larger and truer success; to be willing to accept suffering and to diminish unnecessary suffering; to be able to nourish compassionate relationships; and to listen for and bow down to the goodness of the larger whole.

Satyana's Principles of Spiritual Activism[ccxlvi]

These principles are a wonderful wisdom resource and are used here with permission. *(Permission needed for use.)*

The following principles emerged from several years' work with social change leaders in Satyana's Leading with Spirit program. Any attempt to articulate such principles is clearly fraught with peril. We offer these not as definitive truths, but rather as key learnings and guidelines that, taken together, comprise a useful framework for "spiritual activism."

1. Transformation of motivation from anger/fear/despair to compassion/love/purpose.

This is a vital challenge for today's social change movement. This is not to deny the noble emotion of appropriate anger or outrage in the face of social injustice. Rather, this entails a crucial shift from fighting against evil to working for love, and the long-term results are very different, even if the outer activities appear virtually identical. Action follows Being, as the Sufi saying goes. Thus "a positive future cannot emerge from the mind of anger and despair" (Dalai Lama)

2. Non-attachment to outcome.

This is difficult to put into practice yet, to the extent that we are attached to the results of our work, we rise and fall with our successes and failures—a sure path to burnout. Hold a clear intention and let go of the outcome—recognizing that a larger wisdom is always operating. As Gandhi said, "the victory is in the doing," not the results. Also, remain flexible in the face of changing circumstances: "Planning is invaluable, but plans are useless." (Churchill)

3. Integrity is your protection.

If your work has integrity, this will tend to protect you from negative energy and circumstances. You can often sidestep negative energy from others by becoming "transparent" to it, allowing it to pass through you with no adverse effect on you. This is a consciousness practice that might be called "psychic aikido."

4. Integrity in means and ends.

Integrity in means cultivates integrity in the fruit of one's work. A noble goal cannot be achieved utilizing ignoble means.

5. You are unique. Find and fulfill your true calling.

"It is better to tread your own path, however humbly, than that of another, however successfully." (Bhagavad Gita)

6. Love thine enemy. Or at least, have compassion for them.

This is a vital challenge for our times. This does not mean indulging falsehood or corruption. It means moving from "us/them" thinking to "we" consciousness, from separation to cooperation, recognizing that we human beings are ultimately far more alike than we are different. This is challenging in situations with people whose views are radically opposed to yours. Be hard on the issues, soft on the people.

7. Your work is for the world, not for you.

In doing service work, you are working for others. The full harvest of your work may not take place in your lifetime, yet your efforts now are making possible a better life for future generations. Let your fulfillment come in gratitude for being called to do this work and from doing it with as much compassion, authenticity, fortitude, and forgiveness as you can muster.

8. Selfless service is a myth. In serving others, we serve our true selves.

"It is in giving that we receive." We are sustained by those we serve, just as we are blessed when we forgive others. As Gandhi says, the practice of satyagraha ("clinging to truth") confers a "matchless and universal power" upon those who practice it. Service work is enlightened self-interest, because it cultivates an expanded sense of self that includes all others.

9. Do not insulate yourself from the pain of the world.

Shielding yourself from heartbreak prevents transformation. Let your heart break open and learn to move in the world with a broken heart. As Gibran says, "Your pain is the medicine by which the physician within heals thyself." When we open ourselves to the pain of the world, we become the medicine that heals the world. This is what Gandhi understood so deeply in his principles of ahimsa and satyagraha. A broken heart becomes an open heart, and genuine transformation begins.

10. What you attend to, you become.

Your essence is pliable. Ultimately you become that which you most deeply focus your attention upon. You reap what you sow, so choose your actions carefully. If you constantly give love, you become love itself.

11. Rely on faith and let go of having to figure it all out.

There are larger "divine" forces at work that we can trust completely without knowing their precise workings or agendas. Faith means trusting the unknown and offering yourself as a vehicle for the intrinsic benevolence of the cosmos. "The first step to wisdom is silence. The second is listening." If you genuinely ask inwardly and listen for guidance, and then follow it carefully—you are working in accord with these larger forces, and you become the instrument for their music.

12. Love creates the form. Not the other way around.

The heart crosses the abyss that the mind creates and operates at depths unknown to the mind. Don't get trapped by "pessimism concerning human nature that is not balanced by an optimism concerning divine nature, or you will overlook the cure of grace." (Martin Luther King) Let your heart's love infuse your work and you cannot fail, though your dreams may manifest in ways different from what you imagine.

©Satyana Institute.

"[A] leading evolutionary biologist affirmed [that] 'Recent evidence for directional trends in evolution involve increases in empathy, affectionate attachment, and inter-subjective awareness.' Maybe, just maybe, after three and a half billion years of scrambling, clambering ascent, it's survival of the kindest from here on out." —Marc Barasch

Self-Study Practice:

Please notice and write down three things that resource you spiritually.

1.
2.
3.

What sentences would you give to name your vertical and horizontal purposes?

Now notice how well you are flying with both wings outstretched. Is any wing underdeveloped?

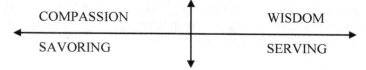

COMPASSION   WISDOM

SAVORING   SERVING

Appendix
U. N. Universal Declaration of Human Rights

On December 10, 1948, the General Assembly of the United Nations adopted a Universal Declaration of Human Rights.

This remarkable document is an ultimate expression of the right use of power. May we someday live up to it. I have summarized it here.

Article 1. All human beings are born free and equal in dignity and rights. They are endowed with reason and conscience and should act towards one another in a spirit of brotherhood.

Article 2. Everyone is entitled to all the rights and freedoms set forth in this Declaration, without distinction of any kind, such as race, colour, sex, language, religion, political or other opinion, national or social origin, property, birth or other status. (omitted second paragraph)

Article 3. Everyone has the right to life, liberty and security of person.

Article 4. No one shall be held in slavery or servitude; slavery and the slave trade shall be prohibited in all their forms.

Article 5. No one shall be subjected to torture or to cruel, inhuman or degrading treatment or punishment.

Article 6. Everyone has the right to recognition everywhere as a person before the law.

Article 7. All are equal before the law and are entitled without any discrimination to equal protection of the law.

Article 8. Everyone has the right to an effective remedy by the competent national tribunals for acts violating the fundamental rights granted him by the constitution or by law.

Article 9. No one shall be subjected to arbitrary arrest, detention or exile.

Article 10. Everyone is entitled in full equality to a fair and public hearing by an independent and impartial tribunal, in the determination of his rights and obligations and of any criminal charge against him.

Article 11. (1) Everyone charged with a penal offense has the right to be presumed innocent until proved guilty according to law in a public trial at which he has had all the guarantees necessary for his defense. (omitted 2)

Article 12. No one shall be subjected to arbitrary interference with his privacy, family, home or correspondence, nor to attacks upon his honor and reputation. Everyone has the right to the protection of the law against such interference or attacks.

Article 13. (1) Everyone has the right of freedom of movement and residence within the borders of each state. (omitted 2)

Article 14. (1) Everyone has the aright to seek and to enjoy in other countries asylum from persecution. (omitted 2)

Article 15. (1) Everyone has the right to a nationality. (2) No one shall be arbitrarily deprived of his nationality nor denied the right to change his nationality.

Article 16. (1) Men and women of full age, without any limitation due to race, nationality or religion, have the right to marry and to found a family. They are entitled to equal rights as to marriage, during marriage and at its dissolution. (2) Marriage shall be entered into only with the free and full consent of the intending spouses. (omitted 3)

Article 17. (1) Everyone has the right to own property alone as well as in association with others. (2) No one shall be arbitrarily deprived of his property.

Article 18. Everyone has the right to freedom of thought, conscience and religion; this right includes freedom to change his religion or belief, and freedom, either alone or in community with others and in public or private, to manifest his religion or belief in teaching, practice, worship and observance.

Article 19. Everyone has the right of freedom of opinion and expression; this right includes freedom to hold opinions without interference and to see, receive and impart information and ideas through any media and regardless of frontiers.

Article 20. (1) Everyone has the right to freedom of peaceful assembly and association. (2) No one may be compelled to belong to an association.

Article 21. (1) Everyone has the right to take part in the government of his country, directly or through freely chosen representatives. (2) Everyone has the aright of equal access to public service in his country. (3) The will of the people shall be the basis of the authority of government; this will shall be expressed in periodic and genuine elections which shall be by universal and equal suffrage and shall be held by secret vote or by equivalent free voting procedures.

Article 22. Everyone, as a member of society, has the right to social security and is entitled to realization, through national effort and international co-operation and in accordance with the organization and resources of each State, of the economic, social and cultural rights indispensable for his dignity and the free development of his personality.

Article 23. (1) Everyone has the right to work, to free choice of employment, to just and favorable conditions of work and to protection against unemployment. (2) Everyone, without discrimination, has the right to equal pay for equal work. (omitted 3 and 4)

Article 24. Everyone has the right to rest and leisure, including reasonable limitation of working hours and periodic holidays with pay.

Article 25. (1) Everyone has the right to a standard of living adequate for the health and well-being of himself and of his family, including food, clothing, housing and medical care and necessary social services, and the right to security in the even of unemployment, sickness, disability, widowhood, old age or other lack of livelihood in circumstances beyond his control. (omitted 2)

Article 26. (1) Everyone has the right to education. Education shall be free, at least in the elementary and fundamental stages. Elementary education shall be compulsory. Technical and professional education shall be made generally available and higher education shall be equally accessible to all on the basis of merit. (2) Education shall be directed to the full development of the human personality and to the strengthening of respect for human rights and fundamental freedoms. It shall promote understanding, tolerance and friendship among all nations, racial or religious groups, and shall further the activities of the United Nations for the maintenance of peace. (omitted 3)

Article 27. (1) Everyone has the right freely to participate in the cultural life of the community, to enjoy the arts and to share in scientific advancement and its benefits. (omitted 2)

Article 28. Everyone is entitled to a social and international order in which the rights and freedoms set forth in this Declaration can be fully realized.

Article 29. (1) Everyone has duties to the community in which alone the free and full development of his personality is possible. (omitted 2 and 3)

Article 30. Nothing in this Declaration may be interpreted as implying for any State, group or person any right to engage in any activity or to perform any act aimed at the destruction of any of the rights and freedoms set forth herein.

Acknowledgements

Creation is a collaboration and a synthesis. I am so happy to honor and appreciate those who have sourced, influenced, encouraged, and inspired this creative compilation.

I am deeply indebted to my colleagues in the Hakomi Institute with whom I have collaborated on the Hakomi Code of Ethics, Hakomi Grievance Procedure, Ethics component of the Hakomi Training, and the exploration of many organizational and personal power dynamics. In particular, to Ron Kurtz, Alan Davidson, Amina Knowlan, Phil DelPrince, Pat Ogden, Jim Schulman, Devi Records, Nina Cherry, Jon Eisman, Julie Murphy, Sahni Hamilton, Jennifer Mueller, Halko Weiss, Mukara Meredith, Melissa Grace, Deepesh Faucheaux, Karen Blicher, Diana Guth, Maya Shaw Gale, Maci Tater, Charlotte Hansen, Laurie Adato, Leighton Hodges, David Knight, Nancy Evergreen, Philip Humbert.

It is with much gratitude that I honor my fellow Earth Song Weavers and ceremonial dancers for the gifts of love, support, challenge, inspiration that we have given and received over the years. I have been empowered and learned much about the largest context of right use of power—soul work, collaboration, and accountability—from Heather Starsong, James Harvey, Allegra Ahlquist, Terry Keepers, Tom Wing, Tom Daly, Jude Blitz, Terry Cohen, Robert Bellows, Zia Parker, Rajan Kose, Seth Henry, Rhonda Hess, Michael Herrick, Dan Raker, Keith Fairmont, Lorraine Fairmont, Kate Guilford, David Phillips, Ken Robinson, Shelley Wittevrongel.

This whole project would not have come to be were it not for the invitation from the Board of Directors of the International Emissary Organization to serve as a consultant to them on the resolution of some ethics issues, the creation of a grievance process, and education in ethics for their members. This work has developed and evolved in the years since 1995 through their appreciation and encouragement. Thank you to Cliff Penwell, David Reis, Leslie Lanes, Barbara Coffman, Michael Cecil, Judy Morris, Elna Stockton, and to Jed Swift for introducing me to the people at Sunrise Ranch.

Thank you to David Patterson and Amina Knowlan for the words: "ethics is right use of power and influence," to Elizabeth Cogburn for her deep wisdom and encouragement, to Nerina Hendry, Marni Harmony, and Anna Cox for their enduring love and faith, to my parents Robbins and Meg Barstow for their shining example of love and right use of power, to my siblings—David and Linda Barstow, and Dan and Eva Barstow—for their generosity and respect.

Thank you to Terry Keepers for sharing his infinite wisdom about the dynamics of shame. Right Use of Power Facilitators offered their help with various chapters: Magi Cooper, Susan Buckles and Greg Johanson added new perspectives to the Shame chapter. Gratitude to Jaffy Phillips and Kathy Ginn for contributions to the chapters on Self-Care and Touch; to Eleanor Velarde and Karen Workman for assistance with the Sexuality chapter, to Cliff Penwell for help with the Transference chapter, and to Patti Tiberi, Judith Blackburn, and Regina Smith for their valuable input in the Influence, Values, Diversity chapter. To Mukara Meredith for help with the Boundaries chapter and Linda Baird with the Grievance Processes chapter, to Peg Syverson for material about escalators, and to Julie Diamond for input about the shadow and perils of power. Additional Right Use of Power Teachers have offered their support and collaboration in the development of this work: Doug Moorhead, Rich Ireland, Meggan Moorhead, Barb Penningroth.

Enormous gratitude goes to Barbara Cargill for her generous contribution of skillful editing. With humor and precision, she coached: "Absolutely no more adjectives!" To Denise Cote for the cover design and numerous other encouragements. To Ben Levi for his patience, skill and artistic support in teaching me how to do the layout and graphics myself (and fixed everything when I couldn't)! To Linda Barstow for correcting details page by page—excess commas, missing words, places where the words didn't match my intention.

Morning after morning I took the SKIP bus down Broadway to the Boulder Public Library where I sat with my laptop Macintosh computer, at a table overlooking Boulder Creek embedded in the changing seasons. The folks at the library created a space free from interruption. Susanna Block, owner of the coffee shop on the library bridge greeted me, tracked my progress, and made me an uncountable number of cups of "haf' caf' mocha with whip" each cup representing at least two hours of work.

About the Author: Dr. Cedar Barstow, M.Ed., C.H.T., D.P.I

I am a one who cares deeply about the right and skillful use of power and influence in the service of person, community, and world.

I work as a Trainer for the Hakomi Institute providing training in the Hakomi Method of body inclusive, mindfulness-based psychotherapy. I am a consultant and teacher on ethics issues and have been designing and developing the ethics approach in this book since 1994. My writing background includes books and articles on women and art expression, massage and counseling with seniors, women and independence, psychotherapy, spirituality, a chapter in *Fire From Heaven: Contemporary Ritual Traditions,* compiled by Ruth Inge Heinz. I graduated in 1966 from Earlham College and received a Master of Education degree from Northeastern University and a degree of Doctor of Psychosocial Intervention from The Parkmore Institute in 2017. I have been associated with the Hakomi Institute since 1981 in numerous capacities including Therapist and Trainer, Ethics Committee Advisor, Managing Editor of the Hakomi Forum, Administrative Director, Librarian, and Board of Directors. I live in a co-operative household in Boulder Colorado and teach ethics and Hakomi Psychotherapy, nationally and internationally.

My most significant experiences in skillful use of power have come through participation in several circles.

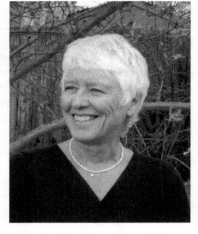

• As one of 12 ceremonial dance weavers, we supported and taught each other skillful use of power in ceremony by sharing the leadership and refining our abilities in giving sometimes hard to hear authentic feedback. We made mistakes, talked about them, experimented with something new, refined the new, accumulated individual and group wisdom, and loved each other. We met monthly for five years.

• As a Hakomi Therapist and Trainer, my concern about the right use of power was focused through personal experiences into being one of the architects of the Hakomi Institute's Code of Ethics, Grievance Process, and ethics component to be taught in each Hakomi Training. The Code of Ethics and the Grievance Process emphasize an ethic of care by attempting the resolution of complaints through effective communication, mediation, appropriate consequences, and education.

• I had the privilege of serving as a consultant to a number of organizations in need of help in effectively attending to misuse of power issues. My recommendations to them cover a broad spectrum: writing a code of ethics; developing an education and repair-based grievance process; guidance and training for leaders; training in making an effective apology and resolving conflict; offering therapy to those who requested it for healing; ethics training for health care practitioners; men's and women's groups dealing with sexual differences in response to, and use of, power; and a series of community meetings on right and skillful use of power and resolution of conflict within relationship.

•   As a member of the Hakomi International Ethics Committee, I have helped shape and refine the ethical grievance process with its focus on resolution and education. I served on the Ethics Committee for the United States Association of Body Psychotherapists, drafting an innovative code of ethics document that includes a section on the ethical use of touch in psychotherapy.

•   My interest in ethics has now expanded beyond ethics for health care practitioners. I see right and skillful use of power as a life-long soul work that is essential for each of us to engage ourselves in. When you are empowered in the best use of your gifts, you can answer yes to the three life questions: Have you lived wisely, have you loved well, and have you contributed? There is so much more to be learned about the conscious use of personal and positional power. How can we use power in the service of person, community and world? This question takes us into realms of right use of power in relation to the earth, in relation to diversity, in relation to governance, in relation to justice. Millions of people, and thousands of organizations pour time, passion, and wisdom into empowered and empowering socially conscious work. With honor and gratitude, I wish this ethics approach to be one more vector in the cause of empowerment and evolved consciousness.

Other Books by Cedar Barstow

Seeds: A Collection of Art by Women Friends, Many Realms Publishing: 1976

Tending Body and Spirit: Massage and Counseling with Elders, Many Realms Publishing: 1985

Chapter 16, Earth Song, in *The Nature and Function of Rituals: Fire from Heaven*, edited by Ruth-Inge Heinze, Bergin & Garvey: 2000

Right Use of Power: Ethics for the Helping Professions, Many Realms Publishing: 2002 (A complete manual for teaching the Right Use of Power ethics approach)

Living in the Power Zone: How Right Use of Power Can Transform Your Relationships, co-authored with Dr. Reynold Feldman, Many Realms Publishing: 2013

Chapter 13, Ethics: Right Use of Power, in *Hakomi Mindfulness-Centered Somatic Psychotherapy: A Comprehensive Guide to Theory and Practice*, edited by Halko Weiss, Greg Johanson, Lorena Monda, W.W. Norton & Company: 2015.

Related Reading

Arrien, Angeles, *The Four- Fold Way: Walking the Paths of the Warrior, Healer, Teacher, Visionary,* Harper Collins: 1993

Barasch, Marc Ian, *Field Notes on the Compassionate Life: A Search for the Soul of Kindness*, Rodale: 2005

Beck, Don and Cowan, Christopher, *Spiral Dynamics: Mastering Values, Leadership, and Change,* Blackwell Publishing: 1996

Benjamin, Ben E., PhD and Sohnen-Moe, Cherie, *The Ethics of Touch.* To order: 1-800-786-4774, or www.sohnen-moe.com

Brooke, Melody, *Cycles of the Heart: A way out of the egocentrism of everyday life,* www.melodybrooke.com: 2006

Brown, G. Scott, *Active Peace: A Mindful Path to a Nonviolent World,* Collins Foundation Press: 2016

Byock, Ira, *The Four Things that Matter Most: A Book About Living,* Atria Books: 2014

Cain, Susan, *Quiet: The Power of Introverts in a World that Can't Stop Talking,* Crown Publishers, New York: 2012

Chapman, Troy K., *Stepping Up: Wholeness Ethics for Prisoners and Those Who Care About Them*, The Whole Way Press: 2011

Chrislip, David D. and O'Malley, Ed, *For the Common Good: Redefining Civic Leadership*, KLC Press: 2013

Corey, G., Corey, M., and Callanan, P., *Issues and Ethics in the Helping Professions, (5th Addition)* Pacific Grove, CA: Books/Cole.

Cornelius, Helena, and Faire, Shoshana, *Everyone Can Win: Responding to Conflict Constructively,* Simon and Schuster, Australia: 2006

Cox, Anna, for newsletter and inspirational messages *www.compassionworksforall.org*

Diamond, Julie; *Power: A User's Guide,* BellySong Press: 2016

Fisher, Roger; Ury, William; Patton, Bruce, *Getting to Yes*, Penguin Books, 1983

Four Worlds Development Project, *The Sacred Tree, Special Edition,* 1988

Fuller, Robert, *Somebodies and Nobodies: Overcoming the Abuse of Rank,* New Society Publishers: 2003

Gerzon, Mark, *Leading Beyond Borders: Thinking Globally & Acting Locally for a Just, Sustainable World*, www.mediatorsfoundation.org: 2004

Hawkins, David, *Power Vs. Force: The Hidden Determinants of Human Behavior*, Hay House: 2002

Halberstam, Joshua, *Everyday Ethics: Inspired Solutions to Real-Life Dilemmas,* Penguin Books: 1993

Hover-Kramer, Dorothea, *Creating Right Relationships: A Practical Guide to Ethics in Energy Therapie*s, www.midgemurphy.com: 2006

Hunter, Mic and Struve, Jim, *The Ethical Use of Touch in Psychotherapy*, Sage Publications: 1998

Jackson, Hildur, Ed., *Creating Harmony: Conflict Resolution in Community*, Permanent Publications: 1999

Johnson, Barry, *Polarity Management: Identifying and Managing Unsolvable Problems,* HRD Press: 1996

Kador, John, *Effective Apology: Mending Fences, Building Bridges, and Restoring Trust*, Berrett Koehler: 2009

Karen, Robert, *Shame,* The Atlantic Monthly, February 1992

Kidder, Rushworth, *Shared Values for a Troubled World: Conversations with Men and Women of Conscience*, Jossey-Bass: 1994

Kurtz, Ron, *Body Centered Psychotherapy, The Hakomi Method,* Life Rhythm: 1990

Lakoff, George, *Don't Think of an Elephant*, Chelsea Green: 2004

Lederach, John Paul, *The Little Book of Conflict Transformation*, Good Books: 2003

Leonard, Sam, *Mediation: The Step-by-Step Guide for Dispute Resolvers,* Evanston Publishing, Inc., Evanston, IL: 1994

Matousek, Mark, *Ethical Wisdom: What Makes Us Good*, Doubleday, 2011

May, John, *Explorations in Ethics for Missouri Counselors: 2000*. To purchase: John May, (314) 822-7972, mayway@earthlink.net

McIntosh, Nina, *The Educated Heart, Professional Guidelines for Massage Therapists, Bodyworkers, and Movement Teachers*: 1999, Decatur Bainbridge Press (877) 327-0600

Moore, Christopher W., *The Mediation Process: Practical Strategies for Resolving Conflict,* Jossey-Bass Publishers, San Francisco: 1986

Phillips, Jaffy, *Somatic Tracking Skills in Assessment for the Use of Touch in Psychotherapy*, unpublished Masters Thesis, Naropa University: 2002

Pope, Kenneth S. and Bouhoutsos, Jacqueline C., *Sexual Intimacy Between Therapists and Patients*, Greenwood: 1988

Pope and Vasquez, *Ethics in Psychotherapy and Counseling*. Jossey-Bass: 1991

Popov, Linda Kavelin, *The Family Virtues Guide, Simple Ways to Bring Out the Best in Our Children and Ourselves,* Plume: 1997

Primack, Joel and Abrams, Mary Ellen, *The View from the Center of the Universe: Discovering Our Extraordinary Place in the Cosmos*, Riverhead Books: 2006

Rechtshaffen, Stephen, *Time Shifting*, Doubleday: 1997

Ries, Shauna and Harter, *In Justice, inAccord,* Booklocker: 2012

Rosenberg, Marshall, *We Can Work It Out,* Puddle Dancer Press: 2003

Senge, Peter, Scharmer, C. Otto, Jaworski, Joseph, Flowers, Betty Sue, *Presence, An Exploration of Profound Change in People, Organizations, and Society*. Currency Doubleday: 2004

Snyder, Timothy, *On Tyranny: Twenty Lessons from the Twentieth Century*, Tim Duggan Books: 2017

Snyder, Martha, Snyder, Ross, Sr., Snyder, Ross, Jr. *The Young Child As Person: Toward the Development of a Healthy Conscience*. (available at www.onbecominghuman.com)

Stamm, B. Hudnall, *Secondary Traumatic Stress: Self-Care Issues for Clinicians, Researchers and Educators,* Lutherville, MD: Sidran Press: 1995

Stone, Douglas, Patton, Bruce, Heen, Sheila, *Difficult Conversations: How to Discuss What Matters Most,* Penguin Books: 1999

Taylor, Kylea, *The Ethics of Caring,* Hanford Mead Publishers: 1995

Ury, William, *The Third Side,* Penguin Books: 1999

Van Hoose, William H. and Kottler, Jeffrey A., *Ethical and Legal Issues in Counseling and Psychotherapy*, 1985

Watkins, Jane Magruder, and Mohr, Bernard, *Appreciative Inquiry: Change at the Speed of Imagination,* Jossey-Bass: 2001

Wheatley, Margaret, and Kellner-Rogers, Myron, *A Simpler Way,* Berrett-Koehler Publishers, Inc.: 1996

Wilber, Ken, *Integral Spirituality: A Startling New Role for Religion in the Modern and Postmodern World,* Integral Books: 2006

Endnotes

[i] George Bernard Shaw

[ii] Joseph P. Firmage

[iii] Karen Armstrong, AARP Magazine, March & April, 2005, (author of *The Spiral Staircase: My Climb Out of Darkness*, Knopf, 2004)

[iv] Marc Ian Barasch, *Field Notes on the Compassionate Life: A Search for the Soul of Kindness,* Rodale, 2005"

[v] Stephen Porges, *Neuroception: A Subconscious System for Detecting Threats and Safety,* Zero to Three, 32, pp. 19-24, 2004

[vi] Marc Barasch, Ibid.

[vii] www.drdan.org/handout%2020.htm

[viii] Amina Knowlan, David Patterson, Group Leadership Training lecture, 1994
The term "right use of power" is used in Angeles Arrien's *The Four-Fold Way*, pages 20-22.

[ix] Elizabeth Cogburn, New Song Ceremonial Dance. This form has only been passed down verbally and experientially.

[x] Angeles Arrien, *The Four Fold Way: Walking the Paths of the Warrior, healer, Teacher, Visionary,* Harper Collins, 1993. Use of the Four Fold Way and wording change from "Tell the truth without blame or judgment" to "Tell and hear the truth without shame or blame" with permission of the author.

[xi] Ron Kurtz, *Hakomi Therapy*

[xii] Ken Wilber, *Integral Spirituality*, p. 61

[xiii] Peter Senge, *The Fifth Discipline*

[xiv] *The Sacred Tree*, Four Worlds Development Project, 1988. This book was produced with the encouragement, wisdom, and guidance of over 100 Native cultural leaders across North America.

[xv] Susan Mikesic, written communication

[xvi] Hakomi Institute Code of Ethics Preamble

[xvii] Robert W. Fuller, *Somebodies and Nobodies: Overcoming the Abuse of Rank"*, from an article

[xviii] Marni Harmony, private communication

[xix]Perry London

[xx] Kenneth Pope, Barbara Tabachnick, Patricia Keith-Spiegel, *Ethics of Practice: The Beliefs and Behaviors of Psychologists as Therapists,* www.kspope.com/ethics/research4.php

[xxi]Golann, S. E., Emerging Areas of Ethical Concern, American Psychologist, 24, (1969)
Golan, 1969, p. 454.

[xxii]Good reference: Rebecca A. Clay, *Psychologists helping psychologists: Determining your responsibilities when you believe a colleague may have behaved unethically, October 2012, Vol 43, No. 9,* http://www.apa.org/monitor/2012/10/psychologists.aspx

[xxiii] Kenneth Drude & Michael Lichstein, *Psychologists Use of E-mail with Clients: Some Ethical Considerations,* kspope.com/ethics/email.php

[xxiv] Sara Martin, *The internet's ethical challenges,* APA, July/August 200, Vol. 41, No. 7, www.apa.org/monitor/2010/07-08/internet.aspx

[xxv] Pope, Tabachnick, Keith-Spiegel, op cit #20

[xxvi] Anna Cox, LCSW

[xxvii] Pope and Vasquez

[xxviii] NASW Code of Ethics, from the website

[xxix] NASW ibid.

[xxx] APA Code of Ethics, 1993

[xxxi] Colorado Association of Psychotherapists

[xxxii] Anna Cox, LCSW

[xxxiii] Ofer Zur, http://www.zurinstitute.com/codesofethics_dualrole.html

[xxxiv] Colorado Mental Health Statute

[xxxv] Nina Cherry, edited from teaching materials

[xxxvi] California Board of Behavior Sciences Newsletter, Fall 2005

[xxxvii] Rites of Passage Council, Inc. at www.RitesofPassageCouncil.com

[xxxviii] Stephen Rechtshaffen, *Time Shifting,* Doubleday, 1997

[xxxix] John May, (2000*) Explorations in Ethics for Missouri Counselors*, p. 10.5 (Reprinted by permission of John May)

[xl] Angeles Arrien, talk

[xli] Mark Twain

[xlii] Karla Schmidt, study of psychotherapy grievances in the State of Colorado. 1995

[xliii] Ofer Zur, *The Ethical Eye*, December 28, 2014 http://daily.psychotherapynetworker.org/daily/ethical-issues/the-ethical-eye/

[xliv] Schmidt, ibid

[xlv] 2004-2005 Fiscal year Summary Statistics, California Board of Behavioral Sciences Newsletter Fall 2005

[xlvi] Ofer Zur, *The Ethical Eye*, December 28, 2014 http://daily.psychotherapynetworker.org/daily/ethical-issues/the-ethical-eye/

[xlvii] Colorado Mental Health Boards

[xlviii] Kenneth Pope, Valerie Vetter, *Ethical Dilemmas Encountered by Members of the American Psychological Association: A National Survey*, kspope.com/ethics/ethics2.php

[xlix] Pope and Vetter, op.cit

[l] Rebecca Smith, psychotherapist and Right Use of Power student

[li] Kenneth Pope, Melba Vasquez, *21 Ethical Fallacies: Cognitive Strategies To Justify Unethical Behavior*, kspope.com/ethics/ethicalstandards.php

[lii] Pope and Vasquez, op.cit

[liii] Marc Barasch, op cit.

[liv] Barry LePatner

[lv] The word Self, spelled with a capital S is from Richard Schwartz' *Internal Family Systems* work. Self refers to a person's essence. Being in Self is an undifferentiated, expansive state in which you feel connections to something greater. This concept of Self is referenced throughout.

[lvi] Starhawk

[lvii] Angeles Arrien, *The Four-fold Way*, pp. 22-25

[lviii] Hakomi Institute Code of Ethics, Hakomihq@aol.com

[lix] Barry Johnson, *Polarity Management: Identifying and Managing Unsolvable Problems.*

[lx] Ron Kurtz, personal conversation

[lxi] Marc Barasch, *Field Notes on the Compassionate Life*

[lxii] Marc Barasch, ibid. p. 219

[lxiii] Rocio Aguirre, class discussion

[lxiv] Terry Keepers, personal communication

[lxv] Robert Karen, The Atlantic Monthly, Feb. 1992 *Shame*

[lxvi] Morgan Holford

[lxvii] Stephen Porges, talk: The Hakomi Conference at the Naropa Institute August 2005. See www.Trauma-pages.com

[lxviii] Inge Mula Myllerup, Hakomi Teacher, from a talk to the Louisville, KY Hakomi Training, February 2006

[lxix] Robert Karen, op. cit.

[lxx] Susan Buckles, Right Use of Power teacher, research, 2005

[lxxi] Donald L. Nathanson, *Shame and Pride: Affect, Sex, and the Birth of the Self*, Norton, 1992

[lxxii] Stephen Porges, op. cit

[lxxiii] Charna Rosenholtz, Right Use of Power teacher

[lxxiv] Johan Huizinga, *The Waning of the Middle Ages*

[lxxv] Robert Karen, op. cit. p. 61, citing Norbert Elias

[lxxvi] Amanda Mahan, private conversation

[lxxvii] Amanda Mahan, private conversation

lxxviii Kylea Taylor, *The Ethics of Caring*

lxxix Dorothea Hover-Kramer, *Creating Right Relationships*, p. 119

lxxx Ibid. Kylea Taylor (adapted)

lxxxi Anna Cox, Social Worker, written communication

lxxxii Susan Mikesic, written communication

lxxxiii Kylea Taylor, *The Ethics of Caring*, adapted from page 50 and 54

lxxxiv Stan Grof

lxxxv Anna Cox, ibid.

lxxxvi Greg Johanson, personal conversation

lxxxvii The exception to this prohibition is for trained and legally sanctioned or licensed sexual surrogates.

lxxxviii Jaffy Phillips, "*Using Somatic Tracking Skills in Assessment for Touch in Psychotherapy*"

lxxxix Richard Ireland, Right Use of Power teacher, input to lists in personal communication

xc Kathy Ginn, Right Use of Power teacher, written communication, 2005

xci Barbara Cargill, personal communication

xcii Geib, 1982, and Horton et al., 1995, in Smith et al., 1998

xciii Jim Kepner, personal communication

xciv With input from Virginia Dennehy

xcv Michael J. Tansey, Ph.D., *Sexual Attraction and Phobic Dread in the Countertransference*, Psychoanalytic Dialogues, 1994, p.141

xcvi Kottler and VanHoose

xcvii With the exception of several legal therapeutic modalities: sexual surrogates, sacred intimates....

xcviii Dujovne

xcix Autumn Cole, *Seeds, A Collection of Art by Women Friends*

c This section is based on notes from: Jon Eisman, Fritz Perls, Denis Postle, David Patterson, Watkins

ci UEF is described in depth by Barbara Brennan.

cii Dorothea Hover-Kramer, *Creating Right Relationships: A Practical Guide to Ethics in Energy Therapies*, p. 59

ciii Patterns as described by Watkins

civ Watkins, ibid

cv Cliff Penwell, personal conversation

cvi Dyrian Benz, Hakomi Training lecture

cvii Mukara Meredith, Hakomi Training lecture

cviii Mukara Meredith, ibid

cix John Bradshaw

cx Edited from Joanna Colrain and Kathy Steele

[cxi] Ira Byock, M.D., *The Best Care Possible*, pp. 197-198, used with permission.

[cxii] Rumi

[cxiii] source material unknown

[cxiv] Cornelius, Helena, and Faire, Shoshana, *Everyone Can Win, Responding to Conflict Constructively*, Simon and Schuster, Australia: 2006. pp. 89-90, used with permission

[cxv] edited from Bill Reidler, Global Relationship Centers, Inc. www.grc333.com

[cxvi] John Kador, *Effective Apology: Mending Fences, Building Bridges, and Restoring Trust,* Berrett Koehler: 2009.

[cxvii] John Kador, op cit, p. 124

[cxviii] John Kador, op cit, p. 52

[cxix] Fred Luskin, *Forgive for Good,* as quoted by Vesala Simic, *The Challenge of Forgiveness*, p.32, *Shift: At the Frontiers of Consciousness, Issue 13*

[cxx] Vesala Simic, p. 30, , *Shift: At the Frontiers of Consciousness, Issue 13*

[cxxi] Jack Lavino, personal conversation

[cxxii] Jack Lavino, personal conversation

[cxxiii] Two excellent videos: *The Power of Forgiveness*, Martin Doblmeier, www.firstrunfeatures.com, 2007; and *Pray the Devil Back to Hell*, Abigail Disney and Gini Reticker, www.praythedeveilbacktohell.com, 2008.

[cxxiv] Barney Aldrich, Master carpenter and life coach, private conversation

[cxxv] Credit for this process, which is certainly an embodiment of the Power Spiral, goes to a long and remarkable circular lineage of its own: It came to me from my colleague Kedar Brown, Eco-Psychotherapist in Asheville, N.C., who adapted it from Bedford Combs and Melissa Jones, Couples Therapists in Nashville, TN, who adapted it from the Men's Council Project (Tom Daly) who was inspired by the four directional work of the Earth Song Ceremonial Community of which I have been a member for 25 years.

[cxxvi] Hakomi Ethics Committee, Sunrise Ranch Ethics Committee

[cxxvii] Mukara Meredith, personal conversation

[cxxviii] Marshall Rosenberg, *Beyond Violence,* Shift: At the Frontiers of Consciousness, Dec 2003-Feb 2004

[cxxix] William Ury

[cxxx] Abraham Lincoln

[cxxxi] Moshe Dayan

[cxxxii] Tom Osborn: www.appreciativeinquiry.org;tomosborn@mindspring.com

[cxxxiii] Marshall Rosenberg, op cit.

[cxxxiv] Marshall Rosenberg, op cit.

[cxxxv] William Ury, *The Third Side: Why We Fight and How We Can Stop*

[cxxxvi] Shauna Ries and Susan Harter, *In Justice, In Accord,* Booklocker, 2012

[cxxxvii] Angeles Arrien, taken from talk

cxxxviii Angeles Arrien, op cit.

cxxxix Yvonne Agazarian, personal conversation

cxl Robbins Wolcott Barstow, personal conversation

cxli Edwin Markham

cxlii Angeles Arrien, talk, The Alchemy of Peacebuilding, Praxis Peace Institute Conference, Dubrovnik, Croatia, June 4-11, 2002

cxliii Janet T. Thomas, *Licensing Board Complaints: Minimizing the Impact on the Psychologist's Defense and Clinical Practice*, 2005 http://janettthomas.com/wpjtt/wp-content/uploads/2012/10/LicensingBoardComplaintsJanetTThomas.pdf

cxliv The ethic of justice and ethic of care are terms used by Carol Gilligan to describe the differences in moral development between boys and girls. Men tend to operate from an ethic of justice and women from an ethic of care.

cxlv Review process summarized from Hakomi Institute International Ethics Committee, www.hakomiinstitute.com, and Ridhwan Central Review Committee, www.ridhwan.org/contact

cxlvi Hakomi Institute Ethical Grievance Process: Statement of Purpose

cxlvii Adapted from a Ridhwan School handout

cxlviii This list is from the State of Colorado Grievance Board covering mental health practitioners

cxlixSteve Vinay Gunther, http://depth.net.au/Resources/Who_Minds_the_Minders.pdf

cl Ofer Zur, op cit #42

cli Ofer Zur, op cit #42

clii Karla Schmidt, State of Colorado study of grievances

cliii Deepesh Faucheaux, Cedar Barstow, Jaci Hull, Hakomi Educational materials

cliv Marilyn Morgan, *What are we doing as Psychotherapists?* paper delivered to Hakomi Institute faculty, 2005

clv Marilyn Morgan, ibid.

clvi Dr. David Patterson, edited from lecture

clvii Mukara Meredith, edited from lecture

clviii Angeles Arrien, The Four Fold Path, used with permission.

clix Angeles Arrien, ibid. Wording changes with permission, from original— "Tell the truth without blame or judgment."

clx Gary Snyder, *Turtle Island*

clxi Charley Thweatt, *Stay in My Hea*rt from CD *Angel on My Shoulder,* www.musicangel.com. Original wording: "Stay in my heart, Stand in my strength." Wording change to "Standing in my power, staying in my heart." used with permission.

clxii Amina Knowlan, personal conversation

[clxiii] Eleanor Velarde, Right use of Power teacher, personal communication, 2004

[clxiv] New England Training Institute lecture, 1969

[clxv] Amina Knowlan, personal conversation

[clxvi] Yvonne Agazarian, through participation in a course

[clxvii] Charna Rosenholtz, personal conversation

[clxviii] Amina Knowlan, *Matrix Leadership*

[clxix] Nathan Cobb, *Post Session Survey*, www.nathancobb.com/post-session-survey.html

[clxx] Bruce Lipton, *Biology of Belief*

[clxxi] Richard J. Davidson, Center for Investigating Healthy Minds, www.investigatinghealthyminds.org

[clxxii] *Fostering thankfulness And improving well-being*, March 2015, www.HealthLetter.MayoClinic.com

[clxxiii] Amit Sood, M.D. *The Mayo Clinic Guide to Stress-Free Living*, Lifelong Books, 2013

[clxxiv] Anna Cox, *What's new for April 2015*, monthly newsletter www.compassionworksforall.org

[clxxv] Kathy Ginn, Right Use of Power teacher, makes this distinction

[clxxvi] E.B. White

[clxxvii] Beck Strong, Right Use of Power Teacher, personal communication

[clxxviii] B. Hudnall Stamm (1995) *Secondary Traumatic Stress: Self-Care Issues for Clinicians, Researchers and Educators,* Preface, p.1

[clxxix] Ron Kurtz, op cit.

[clxxx] Anna Dargitz, personal communication

[clxxxi] Florida Scott Maxwell

[clxxxii] Maya Shaw Gale, mayashawgale@gmail.com

[clxxxiii] Anna Cox, op. cit.

[clxxxiv] Jensen and Bergin, 1988

[clxxxv] Rushworth Kidder: *Shared Values for a Troubled World: Conversations with Men and Women of Conscience*: Jossey-Bass

[clxxxvi] Karen Armstrong, op. cit.

[clxxxvii] Patti Tiberi, Right Use of Power teacher, written private communication

[clxxxviii] Bennett

[clxxxix] Hiromi Willingham, written correspondence, 2014, used with permission

[cxc] Kyle Spencer, *Challenging White Privilege From the Inside*, New York Times, Sunday, February 22, 2015, pp. 24-25

[cxci] Debby Irving, *Waking Up White and Finding Myself in the Story of Race*, Elephant Room Press, 2014

cxcii Peggy McIntosh, White Privilege: *Unpacking the Invisible Knapsack*, Peace and Freedom, July/August 1989.

cxciii Judith Blackburn, private conversation

cxciv Julie Diamond, *Power: A User's Guide*, bellysongpress.com, 2016

cxcv Patti Tiberi op. cit

cxcvi Dacher Keltner, from *Greater Good* magazine, Volume IV, Issue 3

cxcvii Pepi Diaz-Salazar, Right Use of Power Teacher, personal communication

cxcviii Mark Gerzon, *Leading Beyond Borders*, summarized from the book. For more information, go to www.mediatorsfoundation.org

cxcix Dacher Keltner, from *Greater Good* magazine, Volume IV, Issue 3, and other articles and research. Keltner is an excellent resource for theory and research.

cc Webster's Dictionary

cci Yvonne Agazarian

ccii Will Schutz

cciii Arthur C. Brooks, *The Trick to Being More Virtuous*, New York Times, Nov. 27, 2014, http://nyti.ms/1ynurBQ

cciv Senge, Scharmer, Jaworski, Flowers, Presence: *An Exploration of Profound Change in People, Organizations, and Society*. Doubleday, 2004. pp. 177-180

ccv Genda Eoyang

ccvi Carolyn Raffensperger, Whole Earth, Fall 2002, page 34

ccvii Anna Cox, letter from prisoner printed in Dharma Friends Newsletter

ccviii Ron Kurtz, *Body Centered Psychotherapy: the Hakomi Method*

ccix Joris Lammer, Diederik Stapel, *How Power Influences Moral Thinking*, Journal of Personality and Social Psychology, Vol 97 (2), Aug 2009, 279-289

ccx Gene Hoffman, (written source unknown)

ccxi Maya Shaw Gale, mayashawgale@gmail.com

ccxii Karen Armstrong, *Compassion's Fruit*, AARP Magazine, March and April, 2005

ccxiii Gurumai, talk

ccxiv Gary Zukov

ccxv Barbara Kingsolver

ccxvi Barasch, Mark, op cit.

ccxvii Gandhi

ccxviii Tom Hurley

ccxix Karen Armstrong, op cit.

ccxx Moll and Jordan Grafman, neuroscientists at the National Institutes of Health, from an article by Shankar Vedantam, *The Washington Post*, May 28, 2007 [ccxxi] Karen Armstrong, op cit.

[ccxxii] Maryhelen Snyder, personal conversation about *The Young Child as Person*, Martha, Ross Sr., Ross Jr.

[ccxxiii] Robert Hercz, internet article *Psychopaths Among Us*. Dr. Robert Hare has done research on the nature of psychopathy and developed an instrument called the Psychopathy Checklist which is used to measure psychopathy. Using this instrument, he estimates that 1% of Canadians, exhibit psychopathic behavior. Most of these people are not violent, but about 20% of the inmates in Canadian prisons satisfy the Hare definition of a psychopath and they are responsible for over half of all violent crime.

[ccxxiv] Linda Kavelin and Dan Popov, *The Family Virtues Guide*

[ccxxv] see http://www.ted.com/index.php/pages/view/id/162

[ccxxvi] Rushworth Kidder, *Shared Vaules for a Troubled World: Conversations with Men and Women of Conscience*

[ccxxvii] Lawrence Kohlberg, from a summary by Jerry Schueler

[ccxxviii] Carol Gilligan, *In a Different Voice*

[ccxxix] Ken Wilber, *Integral Spirituality*, page 13

[ccxxx] Ken Wilber, op.cit.

[ccxxxi] Ken Wilber, op.cit., page 20

[ccxxxii] Dacher Keltner, from *Greater Good* magazine, Volume IV, Issue 3

[ccxxxiii] Dacher Keltner, op. cit.

[ccxxxiv] Christopher Boehm, Greater Good magazine, Volume IV, Issue 3

[ccxxxv] Dacher Keltner, op.cit.

[ccxxxvi] Dacher Keltner, op.cit.

[ccxxxvii] Dacher Keltner, op. cit.

[ccxxxviii] Rachel Naomi Remen, *In Service of Life*, Noetic Science Review

[ccxxxix] Rabindranath Tagore

[ccxl] Joanna Macy on "Spirituality and Security"

[ccxli] Gandhi

[ccxlii] Angeles Arrien, talk

[ccxliii] Elizabeth Cogburn

[ccxliv] The Dalai Lama

[ccxlv] Barbara Marx Hubbard, lecture 2015

[ccxlvi] Principles of Spiritual Activism. *Satyana Institute's Principles of Spiritual Activism is not for reprint or publication without the express written consent of the Satyana Institute. For permission, please contact Satyana Institute, info@satyana.org, P.O. Box 17904, Boulder, CO 80308, 303-588-7715, www.satyana.org.*

CPSIA information can be obtained
at www.ICGtesting.com
Printed in the USA
BVHW071941260221
601175BV00001BA/49